BRIEFLY PERFECTLY HUMAN

briefly

PERFECTLY

human

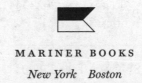

Making an Authentic Life by

Getting Real About the End

Alua Arthur

MARINER BOOKS

New York   Boston

HarperCollins books may be purchased for educational, business, or sales promotional use. For information, please email the Special Markets Department at SPsales@harpercollins.com.

FIRST EDITION

Designed by Chloe Foster

Leaf art © Brandmania / The Noun Project

Library of Congress Cataloging-in-Publication Data

Names: Arthur, Alua, author.
Title: Briefly perfectly human : making an authentic life by getting real about the end / Alua Arthur.
Description: First edition. | New York, NY : Mariner Books, [2024]
Identifiers: LCCN 2023044130 (print) | LCCN 2023044131 (ebook) | ISBN 9780063240032 (hardcover) | ISBN 9780063240063 (paperback) | ISBN 9780063240056 (ebook)
Subjects: LCSH: Arthur, Alua. | Death. | Terminally ill--Care. | Conduct of life.
Classification: LCC HQ1073 .A78 2024 (print) | LCC HQ1073 (ebook) | DDC
  306.9--dc23/eng/20231011
LC record available at https://lccn.loc.gov/2023044130
LC ebook record available at https://lccn.loc.gov/2023044131

ISBN 978-0-06-324003-2

24 25 26 27 28 LBC 8 7 6 5 4

To the too much
To the not enough
To the wanderers
To the aching dreamers
To the perpetual seekers
of nothing to be found

In loving memory: Peter Saint John; Chante Murphy; Angelina Araba Enim; Lindsey Pearlman; Jason Forde; Damain Reeves; Joan Marie; Margo Madji; my paternal grandparents, King Awulae Blay VI and Bozoma Ellimah; my maternal grandparents, JO Evans Enim and Kate Acquah; my thousands of ancestors, many clients, and every person who came before and has already died.

Contents

Author Note

At the crux of my work as a death doula is the element of trust. Clients invite me into their homes and their lives, and with me, they meander through their heartbreaks, proudest moments, greatest joys, sock drawers, and skeletons in the closets. To facilitate this trust, I am morally bound to client confidentiality, and I maintain it to this day. The stories in this book are derived from the most impactful encounters I have had in my work, and the lessons they've taught me live within me still. I did not gain written permission to share experiences of my clients, many of whom are now gone. However, my work with them, and my memories of revelatory connections with them, have endured to the point of bursting.

I use aliases throughout *Briefly Perfectly Human*. To further protect identities, I have changed details and created composites. I combine the experiences of many people with whom I worked closely—including clients who were dying, and those who sought end of life planning consultations and death meditation sessions—with people who simply chose to share their death stories with me in coffee shops, on airplanes, and at parties. It is my intention to create a story in which anyone can find themselves. The experiences we have while dying are universal, yet we feel most alone while journeying through it. I hope these stories show you that we are witnessed, even at the end of our lives. You are seen. You are heard. Your life matters. Your death will too.

BRIEFLY PERFECTLY HUMAN

Chapter 1

A Friend at the End

The car horn blasts, snapping me back to my senses just as I slam my hands on the hood and instinctively pull my body away from the red and yellow taxi. It screeches to a halt an inch before it hits me. Shock waves run through my body like electrical currents, and my breath catches in my throat as the gravity of what almost happened jolts me into the present. Adrenaline has taken over. All the hairs on my body are at attention. Everything is moving in slow motion, like in the *Matrix* when Neo dodges a bullet. I just almost died. And the accident would have been my fault because I wasn't paying attention.

Get it together, Alua! I admonish myself in a familiar way. In the past year I've decided that I don't know how to do anything right. I don't know how to be a happy Legal Aid lawyer anymore. I can't figure out how to feel joy. I don't know how to do life right. I don't even know how to cross a packed street at 8 A.M.

Until that moment, I had never given my death much thought. Yet instantly, I am clear that I don't want to die on the street in Trinidad, Cuba, half drunk, last night's makeup still on my face. My parents would kill me. Being the good Ghanaian daughter I am, I think of the shame I would bring to my family's name by being splattered on the packed street because of my own negligence. I also think about the thong I am wearing underneath my denim shorts. Thongs embarrass my mother. Like most moms, she spoke at length while I was growing up about what kind of underwear I should be found wearing if I were in an accident. This is not the kind she approves of.

The streets pulsate with the business of daily life: mothers taking young children to school, bike taxis herding people to work. The air is filled with honking cabs, and a few horses clickety-clacking as they carry wheat and other goods along the cobblestone streets. I had thought I was outmaneuvering them all by running down the middle of the street, away from the pastel-colored houses. It was a poor choice. With all the chaos, it is no surprise that I didn't see the taxi approaching.

Gathering myself after the near miss, I jump to the sidewalk, next to those who'd stopped to take in the scene I caused. I slow down and move more purposefully, but still too fast. I'm late. Yesenia, a woman I'd met only yesterday, is waiting for me. We'd spent the previous night dancing in a limestone cave like our knee cartilage would last forever, our bodies slick with humidity.

When we met, she was standing in the doorway of her house, squinting and waving as I ran past. I was at the end of an eight-mile jog, heading back to my rented guesthouse. *"Amiga! Amiga!"* she yelled.

When I turned to face her, she began waving more furiously: *"Ven aqui!"*

I slowed and she joined me in the street, a woman in her mid-thirties with heavily kohled eyes. She had seen me earlier and asked why I was running through her town. In fragmented Spanish, I explained that I was visiting Cuba. As a woman who traveled alone a lot, I was familiar with the next question: Where is your husband?

"No hay esposo," I replied. No, nor a boyfriend either. Yes, I had chosen to come alone. And no, there was nothing wrong with me—aside from my poor decision-making, my aimlessness, and the depression coating my brain like a cloudy lacquer finish. How could I translate my need for freedom, my questionable taste in man-child

musicians, my commitment phobia? How would I find the Spanish words to describe a short-lived, six-month marriage that had ended four years earlier, when I could barely understand what happened in English? How could I explain my abject wanderlust, my desire to escape my skin and a life that strangled me? With no clear answer for what I was doing in Cuba, I shrugged.

Yesenia cocked her head to the side, weighing whether or not to fix my man-free problem. Then she offered to hook me up. We'd go to a well-known hot spot later that night, she offered, in the beautiful historic town of Trinidad. I was curious but not optimistic. After three weeks in Cuba, I'd flirted with my share of Cuban men, and noticed how effortlessly they managed to juggle women. Plus, for one of the first times in my life, I was trying not to disappear into a man.

That evening at the appointed hour, I climbed the two crumbling concrete steps into Yesenia's apartment. The wooden door was open and the entrance to her home was covered in a cloth curtain. I could hear the radio blasting the popular Cubaton music I'd grown accustomed to on the island. Yesenia sat me down at her small table with its disintegrating, purple-flowered plastic tablecloth and got to work making me beautiful for the man she'd chosen for me. Apparently he was young, handsome, and would love me in such a way that I would never have to travel alone again. Cuba is for lovers, she reminded me, as she gathered up my locs in a high ponytail and secured it with a bright red scrunchie at the top of my head. The look was 1990s Janet Jackson, circa *Poetic Justice*. She chose a lipstick color that certain generations call "whore red" and enough frosted blue-gray eyeshadow to make the 1980s jealous.

We set out for the club, climbing a steep, rocky dirt path in the dark. I recognized it as the one leading to the Ermita de la Popa church at the top of the hill, from my earlier wanderings in the day. It was pitch black with no humans in sight. As soon as I began to wonder if I'd made a huge mistake, we found a small crowd smoking and chatting beside a large hole in the ground. When we got closer, I could see that the hole was a set of stairs leading down into the earth.

"Espera aquí," Yesenia said.

I was happy to wait on the earth rather than follow her down into it. Yesenia charged forward to see if the spot was open for the night and, moments later, waved her arms for me to join her. She had not told me that we had to descend into hell to find a man. We took a long flight of uneven stone stairs down and entered a maze of tunnels, which eventually opened to a dance floor. Disco Ayala was set deep in a limestone cave one hundred feet underground. Before long, our eyes adjusted to the darkness, and rows of lights, seats, and a dance floor in the middle became clear. It smelled of old cigarettes, sweat, and wet stone. At midnight, the party was just beginning. Surveying the older European male tourists in tight, acid-washed jeans and the young Cuban sex workers dancing alone around them, I figured I was in for a bizarre new experience. Just how I like life.

The night did not disappoint. But the startlingly large man Yesenia had chosen for me did. He was baby-faced but quite tall, with massive muscles, as though his body had matured much faster than his face. He was handsome, but in the way aunties think of their nephews. Carlos and I were not destined to find everlasting love, but we were all entertained by the performances of shirtless Cuban men lying on shards of glass and performing tricks with swords and fire while we listened to Cubaton and Eurotechno.

The brightness of the early morning sky stunned us when we eventually stumbled out, dripping in sweat and pores leaking alcohol. We meandered down the steep hill back to town, laughing, singing, and promising never to forget the night, in broken Spanish and English. As I went off alone to the room I'd rented in a *casa particular*, I realized I still had Yesenia's red scrunchie in my hair. Two hours later, I would need to be up to catch a bus to Santiago de Cuba—a city brimming with vibrant art, music, and the largest population of dark-skinned people on the island.

When my little travel alarm beeped and jerked me awake, I looked at the time and groaned. Then panic set in. I was going to be late for my bus. But first I needed to see Yesenia to thank her and to return her scrunchie, as there were not many new goods in Cuba because of the embargos. I moved as fast as I could to gather my things, which were untidily strewn around the room. My backpack barely closed after my hurried packing. Grabbing a piece of soft, ripe papaya left by my host, I set out to Yesenia's house to return the scrunchie, take her picture, and make it to my bus—all in twenty minutes. It was in this state that the taxi nearly hit me. In the chaos of it all, I reflexively smooshed the piece of papaya in my hand against the hood of the car and felt it squirt up between my fingers. I cursed.

After my near miss with the car, I finally make it to Yesenia's home, clammy and sobered by the experience that, it turns out, will shape the rest of my life. She offers breakfast and another meeting with Carlos. I laugh it off, snap her picture, and thank her, running out the door and promising to keep in touch.

The Viazul bus stop is teeming with people when I arrive, panting, with a couple of minutes to spare. Fumes from the idling buses seep into the doorless ticket office. There are two desks, one with a long line and the other without, and a yellowed, laminated sign hung between them: "*Boletos*." I join the line behind a white woman in her mid-thirties. Her overflowing backpack, army-green windbreaker pants that zip at the knees, and sensible shoes give her away as a fellow traveler. A tattoo of a red quill pen on her right forearm catches my eye.

"Great tattoo," I say.

She smiles. "Yeah, I like to write." *Who gets a tattoo of something they merely like?* I think.

We strike up a conversation. Her name is Jessica.

In deeply accented English (German? French? I know better than to try to guess), Jessica tells me that she is headed to Camaguey, Cuba's third-largest city, on the same bus as I and is surprised that I don't yet have a ticket. Buses are the cheapest way to travel in Cuba, and seats on the Viazul line go quickly. I'm in the wrong line, she informs me. Realizing I'd wasted precious minutes chatting her up, Jessica offers to hold on to my bags and promises with a wink to stall the bus for me. I trust the wink and believe Jessica. Just as I trusted Yesenia enough to follow her into the earth.

While I haggle over ticket prices in a mixture of Spanish and English, I catch sight of Jessica out of the dusty window as she tries to board the bus wearing both of our large travel backpacks. The driver motions for her to take the bags to the underside of the bus. Jessica ignores him. I can hear other people chiming in outside. She ignores them too. I chuckle, recognizing that she is making good on her promise to stall.

Eventually the ticket vendor and I settle on 47 CUC$ for the fare. The ticket should have only cost around 36 CUC$, but I quickly wave it off. Losing 11 CUC$ is not the worst thing my impulsiveness has cost me.

Avoiding the glares of the crowd, I pass through, ashamed when I spot a Cubano who did not get a ticket on the bus and I did—and only because I could pay the higher fare. It stings me, but I barely pause to lament the injustices of my privilege as the bus slowly starts to pull off. I just enjoy the perk, like many who carry privilege do.

I run for the bus, and the driver barely slows down before opening the door for me to jump in. Jessica cheers as I take the last seat next to her in the front row.

"I made an ass out of myself for you!" Jessica giggles, settling in. Besides her shenanigans to hold the bus, turns out she'd convinced someone to switch seats, so that we could sit side by side.

"I know! Why'd you do that?" I ask, still panting. The Viazul's engine rumbles to life again underneath us. Its passenger cabin is strung with Christmas lights and blaring Spanish love songs. Now we are safely underway: two new friends united by the special and strange intimacy of people traveling alone overseas.

Jessica shrugs, giddy. "It worked, didn't it?" She asks what brings me to Cuba. I still don't have a good answer. The truth is less "I'm going through my bucket list" or "I'm a sexy and sassy explorer willing to skirt US travel bans for an adventure," and more "I'm adrift and taking on water in a big dinghy of depression so I took the first float I could find to see if I could save my own life." I've been wandering around the country, riding horses, going on long runs, drinking rum, practicing Spanish, and hoping to find my way back to myself, back into my life, back into my body.

Until this point, life had come relatively easily to me, despite the dark brown skin I wear. I have a tight-knit, supportive family that emigrated from Ghana to the United States, a stellar formal education, a healthy body, and great lovers. I've gone on international trips that most people envy. And, professionally, I work as a Legal Aid lawyer who is supposed to be able to advocate my way into or out of anything. Yet here I am, on a trip for no particular purpose, stuck and deeply unsatisfied.

Back during my senior year of college, when it was time to make big plans, I contemplated how I could be of service. I'm not diplomatic enough to be a politician, even though my dad's politico friends called me Madame President because I'd debate international human rights policies with them as a teenager. I don't have enough patience to be a teacher. I don't want my own kids, and I certainly don't want to be responsible for the care of other people's kids.

The law gave me the most options. So I went to law school because I didn't know what else to do with my one, brief life. Now almost nine years into the profession, I had fumbled my way into a life I despised. I was in the midst of a major depression, a houseguest in my own body. I knew that if I died right then, my last thoughts would be ones of regret.

I spare Jessica the too-soon overshare that I've been told scares people away and give her a nonanswer instead: "I'm seeing what I can see." And I turn the question back on her.

"I'm on a trip around the world," she says. "I started in the States, now I'm in Cuba. Next I'm going to Argentina, Brazil, then South Africa before I go home to Germany."

"And you're on this trip just because?"

Jessica's tone changes and her eyes darken. "Like you said, I'm seeing what I can see." She breaks eye contact for a moment, then continues. "I have uterine cancer. These are the places I want to see in the world before I die."

"Holy shit!" I instantly regret my outburst, but she chuckles. What is the socially acceptable response to this kind of revelation?

I might be sensitive, but that doesn't mean I'm tactful. Never have been. By virtue of naivete, curiosity, boredom, or in this case, lingering tipsiness, I often miss social cues that say a topic of conversation is inappropriate. I forge ahead. "Is this disease going to kill you?"

Jessica's face softens. She looks past my head, across the aisle and out the window. "It might."

"Then what?" I ask. I bite the inside of my lip, instantly wondering if I'd put my big foot too far in my mouth. Again. But I couldn't help myself.

She doesn't skip a beat. "Well, then I guess I'll be dead." We laugh, the deep kind of laughter that quakes with life's fragility.

At thirty-six years old, Jessica is only a couple of years older than I am. We both have illnesses that might kill us if left untreated.

I could die of my depression, I think. Until this point and my near-miss car accident earlier, I hadn't properly considered my own death. The closest I'd come was when teenage AIDS activist Ryan White died in 1990, when I was eleven. That made national news. But this time, it feels . . . different.

I don't know if it's my recent brush with death, the festive setting, or whatever else is stirring inside me, but I begin asking Jessica *really* pointed and personal questions about her life. What will be left undone in her life if cancer kills her? I ask her if she wanted a family. What got in the way of her having one thus far? I ask about her work, her lovers, her dreams, and her sorrows. Finally, I ask her about the end: "What do you think death will be like?"

Jessica tells me this is the first time anyone has asked her these questions or wanted to listen to her talk about her death. Although her oncology program has paired her with a psychiatrist, he is only concerned with how she is living with the disease. He hasn't asked her about dying. Nor have her family and friends made space for her to talk about this fundamental, existential question. She says that whenever she talks about death, they encourage her to have hope, look on the bright side, and focus on healing.

I immediately wonder why we don't make space for people to talk about the questions that lie heaviest on their hearts. Maybe because we think it is too painful to hear. I mean, I'm sparing those closest to me from knowing the depth of my own mental anguish. I don't want to burden them with it. And so my life is full of pretending. I want to protect them from my pain, even as my pain deepens. We all know what's going on, but no one is saying. This strange loop must be infinitely more distressing for an incurably ill person, who cannot afford to pretend that what is happening isn't really happening. When someone is dying, this evasion is a form of existential gaslighting.

It breaks my heart that Jessica is dancing alone with death. I feel called to dance with her in that lonely place, turning and turning in the strange beauty of life, the curiosity of it all. The call is clear and unmistakable. It doesn't require me to be anything other than who I am in the moment. It doesn't require me to think or to know. It only asks me to feel. With all these thoughts rushing through my brain, my next question for Jessica is purely instinctive. "When you look at yourself on your deathbed, who do you see?"

Jessica closes her eyes and considers my question. "I see the scars from my surgeries. I see gray hair. I see my tattoos. Age spots . . . I see a woman who didn't do what she wanted to do." Jessica opens her eyes and tells me how she always wanted to publish a book, to write something for herself. Then her eyes light up: she's had an idea. Maybe she would write a blog about this trip. Maybe that could be her book!

I'm so excited for her that I squeal. Her quill pen tattoo suddenly makes more sense to me. She pulls out her notebook. Her words begin to flow out so fast that she can barely catch up with her own excitement. I watch in joy, knowing something is unfolding, but unclear about exactly what. We drift into amiable silence as she writes, furiously at first and then, after a while, trailing off.

Jessica smiles to herself after one final sentence, then leans against the window. Her eyes flutter and her shoulders soften. The wrist holding the pen slackens, and the pen falls out of her hand. Asleep, she looks so peaceful.

I put on my headphones, beaming. Together, Jessica and I have stumbled onto something that can make her life feel more meaningful—a handle she can hold to pull herself closer to the life she's always envisioned.

Looking out the window toward the cirrocumulus clouds blanketing the countryside, I think about what I want for my life and who I want to be at my death. It's the first time I'm asking myself these questions. I am thirty-four years old.

I realize that the Alua I want to be on my deathbed is a woman who has filled her life cup all the way up and has built a life she feels comfortable leaving. On that bus in Cuba, sitting next to Jessica, I feel far off from being that Alua. I'm a shell of a human, with a mere pinprick of light left inside my body. I feel the heat of shame for not knowing I've been living dead for so long. My insides tighten. But at this moment, having talked to Jessica about death, I feel inches closer to the person I want to be on my deathbed than I did in the moments before.

My iPod shuffles and lands on Bill Withers's "Use Me." I think about how perfect this song is for the life I want to lead. I've always wanted to be of use, useful, used up. That calling led me to my career in legal services, serving low-income communities. But there were parts of me that still weren't being used: my emotional sensitivity, my penchant for the absurd, my love for humanity in all its messiness. A lawyer must see the world in black and white, legal and not legal. I want to bear witness to the full, three-dimensionality of life instead: the confusion, the stubborn love and loyalty, the cognitive dissonance of it all. The both/and.

What would it take to feel fully used up on my deathbed? If I died happy, what would I look like at the end of my life? I see that future self in my head: lifeless hands that held pain and created pleasure, a slack face wrinkled with smile lines and crow's-feet, a lifetime of love shimmering outward from the vessel of my body into the hearts of my family and friends.

Looking around the bus, I take stock of the individuals aboard and wonder what end *they* will meet. There is the bus driver, focused intently on the road ahead. The grouchy woman Jessica convinced to trade seats so that we could sit together. The old man fanning himself with a piece of cardboard. The young mother breastfeeding her child. The child himself.

These people are currently distracted by the daily business of living. One day, they will die. If they sensed the immediacy of life—the preciousness of it, the insignificant significance of it—what would they be doing differently right now? How many unwritten books, undeclared loves, and unfulfilled dreams lie dormant here in these seats and in these bodies? Would they be content dying from the lives they live, or do they hunger for more?

I wonder if they've avoided thinking about dying. I wonder if they've ever had an experience like the one I'm having with Jessica: sitting peacefully with a new friend in the presence of our shared mortality, comparing notes on death with humor, love, and curiosity. Would an experience like this change their lives the way it's already changed mine?

I could be that friend, I think.

I could be that friend for a lot of people.

For the first time since my depression took root, I feel tangible signs of life in my body. Talking to Jessica about death has awakened something within me. Eyes wide. Heart open. Spirit engaged. Pulse audible. Breath measured. Laser-focused. My whole being is present in this moment. Scanning my body, I find no resistance within myself. My natural curiosity, compassion, and ease with difficult emotions has helped Jessica make a little peace with her death, and subsequently, her life. It doesn't require anything more of me other than to be exactly who I am. *Death?* I toss the idea back and forth in my head like a spiky tennis ball, in disbelief. I feel more alive than I have in years. Talk of death is starting to bring me back to life.

After a few more hours of nonstop talking, save a catnap once my hangover finally hit, we reach Camaguey: Jessica's stop on the bus. I've been dreading the moment of her departure and the subsequent seven hours alone on the road to Santiago. I can't tell if the effervescence I feel is because of her or because of my newfound awareness. Jessica stands up and slowly gathers her things. I avoid eye contact. We fumble a goodbye, and she takes a few steps and then turns around abruptly. "What do you think of me coming to Santiago with you?" I yelp a whole body "YES!" and she runs off the bus to make sure her luggage doesn't get pulled off for the Camaguey stop. Then she plops back down beside me.

Jessica and I have no plan, but we have each other. Her caustic sense of humor is a good match for mine. We covet the snacks of the toddler across the aisle, swap horror stories of romance and sex, and make fun of the videos of the Spanish balladeer Camilo Sesto playing on the bus as night falls. The Cuban humidity, bus fumes, our hunger, and the infrequent bathroom stops are inconsequential in our bubble.

Upon reaching Santiago, we scout local stores for Havana Club Añejo 3 Años Rum and a mango juice mixer—as though my liver hasn't had enough—and make it to the guesthouse I'd booked for the night. A middle-aged man greets us on the porch and brings us inside. This *casa particular* is a faded pink, one-story house decorated with aged photos of a woman and lace doilies. Yellowed plastic covers the green velvet furniture. Walking slowly through the house as though on a museum tour, the host shows us around.

He shows us a room with two twin beds and a dresser with a box fan perched upon it. The beds are covered with the kind of flowered quilts one would expect at a grandmother's house. Negotiating a new price for two guests instead of one is easy given our foreigners' currency. Swigs of rum and the Backstreet Boys playing on my iPod eases the evening with my new friend, while cockroaches the size of rodents scurry across the floor. Our luggage sits on the dresser unpacked to avoid our scuttling new friends.

Jessica and I quickly decide we will find a new place to stay tomorrow. We dance for a while, jumping on our beds whenever our insect friends make their appearances. As the night wears on, signs of Jessica's illness become clear. She moves slowly, and her legs and abdomen have built up fluid after the long bus ride. She teaches me how to do lymphatic massage while we talk about where I was when the Berlin Wall came down, how old we were when we got our periods, and how her grandparents helped raise her. Jessica's backpack has a special compartment for the medications she carries—pill bottles of various sizes and colors, daily dispensers with the days of the week printed on them, and loose pills. Medicine galore. And yet here she is living life and bringing her illness along. Living while dying.

Eventually, we settle into the twin beds in this red room with a sun mural on the wall. As I turn out the lights, I hear Jessica turning restlessly in her bed. We laugh that the cockroaches are going to have their own party now. Then she gets serious. "Please don't freak out, okay?" she says in a whisper. I don't say anything, but hold my breath, straining my ears and body to pick up on any clue that I should, in fact, freak out. Was she on the run from the German government? Was she sent by my family to keep an eye on me? Would she try to kill me in my sleep? I'm alone in a room on a little island with someone I've known for only fourteen hours. Maybe I should be worried.

Tentatively, Jessica begins. "Remember when that car almost hit you?"

"Yes," I say slowly, confused as to how she would know about my almost-run-in with the car in Trinidad that began my day. It was before I'd met her at the bus stop. I keep holding my breath.

She continues. "I was in that car."

I don't believe in coincidences. But I do believe in synchronicities and glitches in the matrix. That said, here's what I know now, many years later, in my new life: if not for my "coincidental" encounter with Jessica, I would likely be dead. The burden of living an inauthentic life crowded with societal and cultural expectations was suffocating me. I felt like a failure and couldn't find reasons to continue. Each day I wondered, *What is life for?* Only the thought of reaching the end of my life as the same broken and empty human made space for me to create the type of life I wanted to lead. By envisioning who I wanted to be on my deathbed, I invited life in: the wonder of sustaining thoughtful eye contact with my lover. The joyful tedium of bedazzling roller skates for me and my niece for her tenth birthday party. The inspiration in a job that helps others. The astonishment of my nephew turning eighteen years old in a blink. The awe of birth. The mystery of death.

Societally, we shun conversations about death. Like Jessica's friends and family, who encouraged her to hope for healing instead of considering her end, we pretend we have control over disease and over life. Human beings are funny that way. Our clear inadequacy and powerlessness in the face of death is a reminder of our limitations.

And understandably, that is scary. But the idea of death is a seed. When that seed is carefully tended, life grows like wildflowers in its place. The only thing in our control is how we choose to engage with our mortality once we become aware of it. Cuba is when I became aware. If you are not yet aware, what in the world are you waiting for?

At the time of this writing, Jessica is still alive and in remission. But—spoiler alert—she will eventually die. We all will.

Chapter 2

The Body Always Wins

When I'm called to a bedside, my clients and their families often believe that I know every single thing there is to know about death and dying. But despite the countless hours I have spent with people as they prepare for death, there are many things I will never understand. Who could? Certainly not the scientists, philosophers, or sidewalk preachers among us. They are all still alive. The near-death-experience people? They got to the lobby of death and turned right back around. Death doulas like me? We're still alive too. I can read all the books and get close to death a thousand times over, but without experiencing it firsthand, I'm just as curious and clueless as the next living person. What I *have* observed from the deathbeds of others is that dying is a process of transformation of the body and death marks the end of that transformation. When our time on earth is up, our bodies turn from vibrant, connected vessels animated by something unknown into lifeless, empty matter in the space of a single breath.

Bodies tell our story. At the end of our lives, they give away clues about the type of life we lived. My clients' faces often reveal how they moved through the world. For example, Jonathan's deep furrows in the middle of his brow suggested skepticism and inquisitiveness. He had been an astronomer, and the only bit of flooring visible in his home was the path from his living room to his bedroom. The rest was covered in stacks of glossy science magazines. He stubbornly refused his reading glasses to read them. His constant squinting was visible in his face, even when it was at rest.

A former dancer named Elizabeth, bedbound for three years after multiple knee and hip replacements, had deep smile lines around her mouth with a matching pair around her eyes, stretching upward into her temples and toward the sun. They told of exuberant joy in her life. Even in her final weeks alive, she giggled like she was falling in love.

Frowns, disapproval, and sadness sat in Ernst's jowls. At a diminutive four feet eight inches in height, he was as crotchety as old men come, only allowing me to visit because his daughters insisted. He seemed to delight exclusively in his grandson's obsession with trains, which he also shared. Ernst constantly looked like there was rotting fish in the room unless his grandson was around.

Edward's upper arms, torso, and thighs were covered in tattoos. He was a big-time corporate lawyer who headed up a motorcycle club in the suburbs where he lived. He left his calves and forearms un-inked because of golf vacations with the associates at his firm.

And then there's my body. I hope that when I die, my body says that I danced, enjoyed the warmth of the sun on my face, and loved both squats and french fries.

On May 29, 1978, weighing in at a hefty ten pounds, my body arrived on Earth to play. God bless my mother's body. She'd lived twenty-six years, had a short Afro and a body that had already been inhabited by my sister when I took up residence there. Since her first child was only six months old, she didn't know she was pregnant with me. She didn't believe women could get pregnant while breastfeeding. She was wrong. I was conceived in London but don't want to know too much about that, other than that I traveled in utero to be born in Ghana. Been traveling ever since.

My birth was my first death—from the womb into this world. I changed form. Changed the way I breathe. Changed environments and left the only place I knew thus far—the comfort of my mother's body—much to her delight since I was three weeks late. Or as I like to say, right on time, just not according to scientific projections. This was in Accra, Ghana's capital city, and the only thing to do was be patient till I made my entrance. No Pitocin, no epidurals, no options except to let nature take its course and let my mom's body do what my mom's body would do. I arrived after a long labor on both of our parts. Hers was powered by a meal of Tuo Zaafi (a northern Ghana dish of corn dough, vegetable stew, and meat) while straddling a toilet; mine by a shimmy shake to get these wide shoulders of mine down her birth canal. I was born while the sun was in Gemini and the moon was in Pisces. Gemini was rising on the eastern horizon.

A huge and wide-eyed infant, I grew into a chubby kid. In Ghana being a heavy child is a source of family pride. We call chubby kids *bofti* as a term of endearment. It signifies wealth, health, and good upbringing. And a hefty appetite, which mothers seem to love.

As a child, my namesake, Aunty Alua, my dad's favorite aunt, screams *"Bofti!"* gleefully whenever I approach, trying to pick me up, groaning with delight about how heavy I am. She is elated that my parents have chosen to name a child after her. Fawning all over me and pinching my round cheeks, she rushes me into her home to sneak me candies, cake, and my favorite Muscatella soda, which tastes like cream soda mixed with pineapple and ginger ale. Being in my body as a child, I felt celebrated, wanted, safe, and loved.

When we finally moved to the United States when I was eleven years old, my relationship with my body grew tense. Being chubby was looked down upon here. So was being Black. My body suddenly became reviled, an enemy, something to fear and fix rather than appreciate for the miracle it was. As a preteen, my curves attracted attention I did not want.

Now as an adult, I've found harmony with my body by rooting myself in the mystery of its existence and delighting in its power and grace. I'm no longer trying to rid myself of the little pooch that sits on my lower abdomen through crunches and two-minute planks. Instead, I'm savoring tortilla chips dipped in Nutella and truffle mac 'n' cheese.

I am chubby no more, but still big. Being big is not a choice. I stand five feet ten inches tall, in a deeply melanated, female, shapely, energetic, able, and athletic body. For now. I consider every last one of these attributes to be privileges, despite what the outside world validates. My facial features are strong—razor-sharp cheekbones and unapologetic, wide-gapped front teeth. My collarbones sit prominently, deep enough to hold water. My arms have thick biceps that accompany my child-bearin' hips and malleable hamstrings down below. My long fingers and wide palms can grip a woman's basketball from the top with one hand, despite my delicate and ornately painted nails.

My sturdy legs are marked with scars, big and small—evidence of a lifetime of clumsiness and adventure. And I've got big ole feet that I trip over. All of the bones I've ever broken are in my feet, earning me the nickname Grace, as a joke. (The irony that this nickname is now part of the name of my death doula business, Going with Grace, is not lost on me.)

Sometimes when a stranger hears my voice over the phone, I am called "mister" or "sir," especially in the morning when my voice is deep and husky. I speak with a lisp—putting a little twist on my *s*—which I can't hear except when audio is played back, or when the kids in middle school made fun of me. It's a tongue thrust that speech therapy didn't get rid of. I don't find anything wrong with it. It's just different in America. It would work in Spain.

My hair is dreadlocked and hangs down to the middle of my back.

THE BODY ALWAYS WINS 21

Several of the locs are jazzed up with gold strings, charms, and cowrie shells. I decorate my body heavily, choosing brightly colored clothes, adorning my ears and nose with many piercings, and draping my fingers and wrists with what some would consider an excess of brass and copper jewelry. I scent myself with frankincense and myrrh.

People stare at me wherever I go. Significantly more in Jaffna, Sri Lanka, than in Bedford-Stuyvesant, Brooklyn. But no matter—I'm gonna give them something worth looking at. I'm only here for a small amount of time. So I insist on taking up space in the world, in rooms, in my life, and in my relationships. I wouldn't have it any other way. I am here. This is my body. It is the place I live and also the place where I will die.

In time, my body, like all bodies, will shrivel and deteriorate. I'm already losing collagen in my skin and pigment in my hair follicles, and I need to pee more often than I used to. My cells are having a harder time replenishing the nutrients that come via food and the environment than they did yesterday. My boobs sag and I've fully surrendered to cellulite, even in my arms. I only learned that was a thing after I turned forty and fat started settling in places it hadn't before. Lines are forming around my eyes, and the one in between my eyebrows is deepening. My facial skin feels thinner while the skin around my elbows and knees is thickening. No amount of anti-aging creams or vitamins can stop this bodily process. At this very moment, I am the youngest I will ever be again, and also the oldest I've ever been. I'm human. I was born. I will age. Not aging means I am dead. So for now, I'd rather take glucosamine for my joints and use an eye cream to keep my skin supple.

Day in and day out, we trust our bodies to carry out billions of tasks for us, without much, if any, participation from us. Are you aware of how many breaths you've taken or how many heartbeats have passed while reading these paragraphs? (Around 360 heartbeats and between 60 to 100 breaths, depending on how quickly you read.) Or how much additional sensory information you are receiving at this moment to regulate your temperature? When we get a paper cut, most of us can effortlessly trust that the tiny but painful wound will heal on its own. The body sweats, alchemizes minerals, processes food, creates waste, blinks, releases oil, creates red blood cells . . . you get the point. It works without a thank-you for all the functions it carries out so we can live. We inherently trust the body.

We trust the body to turn us on when sexually aroused and turn us off to go to sleep. Millions of neurons fire when we have a fleeting thought, and we trust our thousands of taste buds to distinguish between sweet and bitter. The body alerts us to something that requires our attention through pain and sends white blood cells into our tissues looking for invasive bacteria and viruses to kill off before they kill us. Without our conscious knowledge, the body alerts us that there is danger nearby by raising hairs on the back of our necks. When there are strong emotions (or an extrasensory perception), the body will contract the muscles that are attached to each hair follicle, causing our skin to raise. We know this as goosebumps. (I call them *juicebumps* because something pretty juicy is normally going on when goosebumps arise.)

The body is our most trustworthy companion. We care for our bodies in many ways, often superficially. We cover our bodies in clothes, we get haircuts, drink fancy water, eat food, shower, and slather on moisturizer. (If you don't, please start. Don't be ashy for the blip of a moment you are alive.) And finally, we rest when we are tired. Science and medicine cannot fix everything. Until the antiagers and the cryonics folks find a work-around, the body will always win.

Ask me how I know.

For nine long weeks in my late thirties, I trained to be a competitive middle-distance runner: 800 meters, 1,500 meters, and the mile. A man I'd met at a park while I was stretching mid–recreational run complimented my physique and form. Thinking he was hitting on me but noting his use of the scientific names for my muscles, I paused. He thought I held promise as a middle-distance runner and since I liked to run anyway, I gave it a shot. He wanted to train me for free to regain some of his former running coach glory. I would be the Rocky to his Mickey. I agreed to meet him each Tuesday for ten-mile runs, Thursday for weight lifting, and Saturday for sprint practice at the track where his former running colleagues trained and where he would show me off.

During the weeks we trained, I was ravenous. I slept almost ten hours every night. My body grew sinewy and ripped. My brain was clear, as was my skin. I could catch a jar falling off a counter before it hit the ground. I felt like a machine and my booty was getting rounder and higher. Wins all around, but especially in the back.

For nine weeks I ran. Every week, I added miles to my feet and knees and ran in short and long bursts hoping to make my race times shorter. In two 5K races, I placed at the top of my age group. Tuesdays burned my lungs, but I could cover the distance. Thursdays burned my muscles, but I could push through the weight. Saturdays I felt like a failure when, during each 400-meter training sprint, my body slowed down significantly after 250 meters. I sweet-talked and yelled at myself to push through: *keep going, KEEP RUNNING GO GO GO ALUA!* I even imagined I was getting chased by someone forcing me to wear high-heeled Crocs—all to no avail. On a track with elite amateur and some professional runners, I would run out of gas and sit down in the middle of the lane. A disappointment to my coach. Despite my Flo-Jo and Rocky dreams, my natural athletic ability and steel will, I could not sprint the full distance.

We changed my lifting schedule. I added more carbohydrates to my diet. I stopped distance running even though that's what I loved. We tried shifting into shorter sprints, but they weren't enjoyable for me. I'd tell my body that it could do anything. But it couldn't sprint past 250 meters. When running at max capacity, my body would shut down at about 300 meters. Mind over matter does not always produce the intended result. My body won.

The mind is powerful. But the mind can't do it all. The mind certainly cannot stop people from dying when the body in which it is rooted is ready. I've known many people who really *want* to live but still die, because the body has reached its end. At some point, the best we can do is listen to it, and trust the workhorse is tired and it is ready to die.

Those of us with privilege can stave off the inevitable for longer: buy the more expensive treatment, see the out-of-network specialty doctor. Likewise, perhaps with focused nutrition, hyperbaric chambers, and gait dissection, I could have run farther. But ultimately, you can't outrun the body you're in, or buy your way out of a sick and dying one.

But let's not talk of our bodies as prisons. In these bodies, we have the privilege of experiencing the magical playground of Earth. Because of our bodies, we get to eat donuts, jump in puddles, smell rare spices, listen to children's laughter, blow bubbles with gum, make art, make flan, and make love. Because we get to live, we get to die. Death does not happen *to* us. It is something that we do. *To die* is an action verb.

I want my body to be as full as the life I lead. I want to stay at home in this body for as long as I am able to ride this spinning blue ball. I recognize now that my earlier depression was an invitation from an empty body to fill it. Constantly seeking and never satiated, I was a hungry ghost for life. My lifetime of hunger for food (I wasn't chubby for nothing) is also my hunger for connection, joy, meaning, and love. These days, I can't make my body small if I want to. I can make it quieter, but I have chosen to live loudly. I have chosen to stand as close to death as I can, by accompanying people to their ends. And each time, in this profound process, I am reminded of the celebration of life and the enormity of our miraculous existence. All because of these amazing bodies we're in.

What will it take for us to fall in love with our bodies? To trust them, honor them, and grant them release when death comes? Because by the time we have reached the end of our lives, our bodies invite us to surrender, having already luxuriated in the rich experiences of the world. All life eventually needs relief from the intricacy of living. Nature does what nature does. It has since time immemorial. Nobody gets out alive.

Chapter 3

Death at Our Heels

My earliest memory of life is of escaping death. It is December 31, 1981. I am three years old. My older sister, Bozoma, is four, and my younger sister, Ahoba, is one. I hold my dad's big hand as he rushes me down the back stairway of the government officials' building where we live in Accra. Normally cool, velvety, steady, and dry, my father's hand is hot and sweaty, gripping mine as though he fears I'll slip away. My toddler legs can't carry me fast enough down the seven flights, so eventually, my father carries me. From over his shoulder, I can see through the glass windows into the courtyard.

The government of Ghana is being overthrown in a military coup. When a plot to overthrow a government fails, the coup plotters are killed for treason. When the plot is successful, the existing government officials and anyone who stands in the opposition's way are the ones who get killed. In both cases, hundreds of people senselessly lose their lives in the midst of riots, mayhem, and anarchy. I am too young to understand it, but the fear of death blankets Accra this morning.

When I close my eyes now, images from this fateful morning remain with me: car doors flung open, belongings hurriedly stuffed inside. Car horns honking, impatient. People rushing about, panicked. The mental pictures feel both vivid and unfamiliar, like stills from someone else's family photo album. It would be years before I even realized where they came from.

Everything I know about that day, apart from these disconnected flashes, I learned secondhand from my parents through conversations about this terrifying moment in their lives. I was an adult by then. It was strange, hearing about our flight and trying to place myself in it. I was there, but I'll never truly know all that I felt. Maybe I was just too young to understand what was happening around me, or maybe this blank spot is the protective cocoon of early childhood trauma. I'll never know. More than anything, I recall the warmth of my father's hand. In the midst of chaos caused by the fear of death, I know I felt calm and safe with him holding on to me.

Whatever its effects on me, the story of the coup belongs to my parents. They were the ones whose bodies bore the weight of that firsthand experience. What follows is their story, or as much of it as they've chosen to share with me, filtered through time, distance, and their own pain.

My father, Dr. Appianda Arthur, was a prominent government official under Ghanaian president Dr. Hilla Limann, who was suddenly no longer the president. If we stayed in our apartment, my father would die. And in all likelihood, so would we. So we rushed down the stairs to get to safety because the elevator was busy with other government officials and their families, also desperate to flee. At thirty-six years old, my dad was a rising star in Ghana's political landscape. He'd earned Ph.D.'s in ethnomusicology and anthropology at Wesleyan University in America (which I would eventually attend) and enjoyed an illustrious career as a lecturer at the University of Ghana (which I also eventually attended—definitely a daddy's girl).

Additionally, my father represented Nzema East in the Western Region of Ghana as a member of Parliament; he was on the committee overseeing the office of the President, and sometimes he traveled as part of President Hilla Limann's entourage. The Limann administration had only been in power for a little over two years, and now the government was being overthrown by J. J. Rawlings, a notoriously violent figure in Ghana's political history. It was a perilous time for our family.

My mother, a Fante woman named Aba Enim, who worked as a fashion model in London before marrying my father, hadn't signed up for any of this. There is a picture of her tucked away in her things that I've only seen once from before she was a mom; close-cropped Afro, denim booty shorts, a crocheted bikini top, and platform shoes—as sexy and badass a woman as the 1970s ever made. There's a cigarette dangling out of one hand and a dark beverage in a tumbler in the other, a record player behind her. But now, her life was different. She'd been sewing cushion covers for a furniture company because we needed the extra money. A career in politics isn't particularly lucrative in Ghana.

The marriage was a smart move for my father. Just as my mother's modeling and fashion design career had started to blossom, he had snagged her and taken her to the United States, where he finished his doctorate degrees. She never wanted to be a working mom to three girls under five. She certainly didn't want to be frantically clutching them all and running for her life in her nightgown from a gang of armed insurrectionists.

After the 7 A.M. official announcement came over the radio that the government had been overthrown and all those who worked for the government should immediately surrender or risk arrest and execution, my parents rushed us to my uncle Paa Kwesi's house. My mom forgot my little sister's breakfast porridge. This seemed a small oversight, but turned into an unspeakable terror when she tried to retrieve it. In recounting this harrowing trip to me years later, the details proved too much for even my iron-willed mom to convey fully. She could only relay the story in slivers. My heart breaks for what she endured. The grace with which she wears this quiet pain looks, to me, like the epitome of strength.

A few days after the coup, my father decided to turn himself in rather than risk getting caught. Soberly, he and his government friends got into a van that drove them to the Nsawam prison on the outskirts of Accra. When my father described this moment to me over the phone recently, I was touched to hear his voice constricting. "Bozoma asked me if I'd be back for her birthday in three weeks' time," he told me. "She would be turning five. I couldn't tell her that I didn't know if I'd ever see her again. I wept." My father is not the type to tear up; his difficulty in relaying this moment to me, even forty years later, showed me just how deep the wounds were.

As he told it, a parade of arrogant opposition soldiers greeted him with kicks, taunts, slaps, and the butts of their guns. For the next five months, he sat in a corner of the prison reserved for those whose fates were still undecided. During that time, he found a Gideon Bible and decided to dedicate his life to the service of God. His heart filled, and he was given over to a singular purpose. Whatever else was going on in my father's heart in that jail cell—fear, anger, anxiety, boredom, confusion—I know that his conversion was total and sincere.

When it was time for my father to be tried before a military tribunal for his "offenses," he told the judges about his newfound commitment to God and promised to spread God's love if he was released. They laughed, having already sentenced his government friends to thirty or forty years for "corruption."

While my father was in prison, my mom also found Jesus. Her conversion happened at a revival in Accra. If anything, hers was even more unlikely than his: her faith was usually only observed a couple of times a year during weddings or funerals. But I see how being a single mom of three with a husband in prison would drive anyone to seek out a higher power. Desperation is often fertile soil for faith.

One saving grace during this time was that my parents had grown close to Americans at the US embassy in Ghana after their time in the States. Those relationships made it easier for my mother to implore her embassy friends to keep a watchful eye on my father's situation, as the United States had eyes on the political unrest in Ghana. For weeks and weeks, my mother toiled, unsure of whether she would ever be reunited with her husband again.

After six months, remarkably, the prison officials took my father seriously and they decided to release him in early May, just in time for my fourth birthday. My parents' Christian faith and prayer had proved itself, and their reunion was so exultant that they conceived a fourth child. My sisters and I secretly wished for a brother.

After my father's release, an old classmate of his, Chris Weaver, worked with the US embassy to help secure our travel to the United States. My dad stayed behind because his passport had been seized. Off my mother, sisters, and I went to Bethesda, Maryland, to live with "Uncle Chris," while my father sorted out his escape from Ghana. Pregnant and with three very small children, my mother boarded the plane with us and settled in for the long flight. I was oblivious to the gravity of the situation, of course, and have always been unable to sit still for long. I remember walking up and down the aisles of our international flights, making friends with fellow passengers.

Upon arrival, my mom was alone in a country in which she'd only spent a few years. Falling apart would have been an easy option for her. But it just isn't in her DNA. To hear her tell it, she carried the weight effortlessly: expat wife and suddenly single mother, a warrior in love. By the time she arrived in Bethesda, she was faithful to and well versed in Christianity and actively sought out community, as she waited patiently for my father's return. She found it in the yellow pages: the First Baptist Church of Bethesda. One Sunday she enrolled us in the church preschool and got a job there. It was only after persistent prodding from me that she revealed she often cried in the bathroom by herself, usually with me or one of my sisters banging at the door.

After some serious serendipity and a laborious route out of Ghana, guided by farmers by day and fishermen by night, my father made it to the Ivory Coast and eventually into Liberia. There, he was classified as a political refugee and obtained an international passport, which allowed him to join us in Maryland. Six months after we left, he was safe and reconnected with us, but the road ahead remained uncertain.

In Maryland, we settled into our first full-time home in America. I have few memories of the years in Maryland, but all of them are of safety and family: A babysitter put mascara on me. I decided it made my eyelashes too long, so I cut them, to the horror of the babysitter, who had to explain why a young child took scissors to her eyes under her watch. I remember my fifth birthday, and the delicious chocolate cake that I reluctantly shared with Ahoba, who turned three at the beginning of *my* birthday month. For the occasion, my mother made us matching outfits out of Ghanaian fabric. We wore a lot of matching homemade clothes in childhood. I thought they were endlessly cool, but my classmates often disagreed. With the supreme confidence of a five-year-old, I shrugged it off. (Adolescence was another story.) We were outsiders, anyway. And my parents came home from the hospital with yet another girl—my baby sister, Aba. My sisters and I were sorely disappointed. I remember asking my mom to take her back, but today, I could not imagine anyone but her. She grounds me. Aba completed our family.

For years, we were missionaries and political refugees, bouncing around the planet while my dad took jobs preaching and spreading the gospel of Jesus. Wherever we went, the six of us got on the stage. My father as the visiting pastor, his beautiful wife, and his four girls in matching outfits. We'd smile for pictures, wave, and head off to the next church the following Sunday. For longer stints, we spent time in Pasadena, California, while my dad taught at Fuller Theological Seminary. We lived in Nairobi. We even traveled back to Ghana for a few years, as my father headed up the African regional office of Prison Fellowship International, sharing his story of redemption in prisons across the continent. After my dad served his initial prison term, his offenses were erased, and we were allowed in the country safely. My father's work often sent him on international travel, which gave my mother a chance to see other parts of the world and spend time alone with him when my sisters and I stayed behind. Fellow missionaries and family friends watched my rowdy bunch of sisters and me in my parents' absence, and when Mom and Dad came back, they returned bearing gifts.

From Manila, they brought multicolored jelly sandals. To this day, in my mind, the Philippines is the land full of glittery rubber shoes. When my dad returned from Australia, he brought back a metal trunk full of goodies, including a boomerang. I remember him throwing the boomerang in the house and my mom yelling at him, because she knew I would run after it inside the house. I did, slicing my right calf on the corner of the metal trunk. Today, the five-inch-long scar still reminds me of all that has been possible for my family, even in the face of chaos.

I was angry for a long time. For most of my adolescence and early adulthood, I believed that J. J. Rawlings and his soldiers stole Ghana from me that New Year's Eve. Had he and his forces never overthrown the government, I might have grown up in a country with people who looked like me, ate my food, spoke my language. I could've dated people with whom I didn't have to navigate cultural differences. I might have gone every year to Kundum, a festival in my dad's region, or might have learned to bargain in Accra's markets. I might have grown up eating my favorite snack of deep-fried ripe plantain rolled in pepper, ginger, and salt—also known as kelewele.

The coup meant that I was forced into life as an outsider wherever I went. I was never Ghanaian enough by virtue of not being raised there, and never American enough due to my Ghanaian heritage. I never know how to answer the question "Where are you from?" Is the answer where I was born? Where my parents are from? Where I was raised? Or where I live? Or where I lay my head? "Home" has always been a fleeting concept for me, and I've had to learn to cultivate it in my body.

Sometimes I've wondered if the coup, and all the consequences that unfolded from it, molded me in ways I may never fully understand. My earliest memory is of thrilling, death-defying flight. Does this help explain the perpetual unrest living in my spirit, my never-ending yearning for adventure? Maybe that fateful flight down the back steps in Ghana rewired my little brain, and I was forever afterward drawn to peak experiences.

It would certainly track. I've struggled all my life with a near-pathological fear of boredom. I don't think of myself as a thrill seeker, but I'm certainly an experience junkie. Falling in love. Music festivals. Psychedelics. Heartbreak. Adventure, dopamine, oxytocin. Flood my body with chemicals that make me feel alive, please.

As a child, I complained constantly of being bored. "Go read a book," my parents would say, exasperated, to which I'd say, "I read them all." (I had.) I took everything apart—I unraveled blankets, disassembled remote controls. I was driven by an insatiable need to figure out *why* things were the way they were. School was torture, as were the rote recitals of the lessons, the complete lack of questioning. Soon I experienced the same frustration in the lack of questioning of Christianity. Sitting still was a punishment that I chafed against by constantly talking to the people next to me, by constantly moving. Boredom was a force pinning me down; I wouldn't let it get me.

Even more than the scariest feelings—trauma, loss, terror, grief—I've always feared monotony. Maybe the flight path our family took across the globe has something to do with that. Or maybe I was destined to be a nosy, bright, curious, awkward, fidgety, and sensitive kid, no matter where I was born.

Whatever the case, the coup arrived in our lives unexpectedly. When the unexpected comes in to rob us of something we treasure, it can also bring about incredible opportunity. Just like death itself.

The truth is that the coup, and all the death it brought, created opportunity for my family. We are extremely close. No matter where I go or have ever been, my sisters remain my best friends, but we're not without our challenges. We grew up packed in like sardines—four kids in six years—so naturally we wanted to kill each other occasionally, but we also would want to kill anyone who so much as looked at one of us wrong. I belong with them. As adults, our deep sister-bond feeds and nurtures me in a way that would not have been possible without the constantly changing backdrop of our childhoods. And since we're all tall with big feet and varied senses of style, I've got three additional wardrobes and shoe closets to peruse. If we had stayed in Ghana, we would have never grown to be the women we are today. Who else but my sisters can understand the implications of our childhoods, the all-night Christian revivals, constant travel, Ghanaian food school lunches, and our secret adolescent rebellion against Christianity?

So yes, death can be a thief. But death is also what brings life. Dead leaves fall from the trees and nurture the soil. People die and make space for new ones to be born and populate Earth. Our aging cells continually die off so that the new ones can thrive. When I look back at the life I've lived, I can appreciate the synchronicity of it all.

In those capricious times, my sisters and I did not know of the struggles my parents faced to provide for us while holding on to their mission work. Despite what they were going through, my parents decided that girls becoming women need stability. So in 1989, we moved for the last time as a family, settling in Colorado Springs. It is the world's center of the Evangelical Christian movement—white, military, and highly conservative. Eventually, in 2006, my parents divorced, selling the house they built with a finished basement just for my sisters and our friends. We were scattered to the winds but somehow also still one, bonds forged by blood, death, and experience.

Little deaths abounded each time we said goodbye to a house (the addresses of which I will always remember), friends (names of which I've mostly forgotten), customs, rituals, and familiarity. We were changed by each experience but quickly learned new places, new people, new foods, new ways. Today, we are a mosaic of every place we've ever been, a reflection of those we've ever met, and a tapestry of who has touched us.

We are a tight-knit crew: my thoughtful, resilient, worldly, charismatic parents, and four bright and bold daughters—same shine, different sparkle. We survived. We move about the world as one unit where nothing—*nothing*—could infiltrate our circle. That is, until Bozoma met Peter, and he became our family too.

Chapter 4

Peter

I wish I'd understood when he said he was tired that he meant he was *life* tired. He was living-in-a-sick-body tired. He was ready-to-die tired. I didn't understand. Peter murmured something I couldn't hear, so I leaned in closer. His voice was weak, given the tumors that had been growing in his throat and on his vocal cords for months.

"What did you say?"

"I'm tired." He grunted. His right eye searched for mine. His other eye was covered by a patch because it had started to wander in his head as his cancer progressed and attacked the muscles that controlled it.

"Then rest, okay? Rest." I smiled and very gently patted his leg. The corners of his mouth barely turned up under the weight of his exhaustion. He couldn't feign a smile. With a quick kiss on his oily forehead, I gathered my things and said good night to my sister Bozoma, my mother, and Peter's parents, while my four-year-old niece, Lael, also said her goodbyes. Without a second look back, we left the hospital room. Those were the last words my brother-in-law Peter ever said to me. He slipped into unconsciousness that night and died three days later. Peter taught me how to be a death doula. He also taught me that you never quite heal from the pain of loss. You just learn to live with it.

In 2001, my older sister, Bozoma, started talking about a guy she'd met in the cafeteria at work. She worked at Spike DDB, a subset of the DDB advertising agency headed by Spike Lee, as a junior account executive, and Peter worked for DDB on the creative side. Over the phone, she told me of this man who had wined, dined, and flower-showered her. As the weeks turned into months, it was clear that Peter Saint John was going to stick around.

Peter was gregarious, ambitious, funny, and silly. At six-four, socially conservative, and Irish-Italian from Boston, he was also unlike anyone in my social circles. His sense of style was entirely absent, except for his taste in leather jackets. He wore tube socks with loafers, for God's sake. We butted heads about everything: the death penalty, making career decisions from passion, vegetarianism. Bozoma refereed. The social justice warrior in me made him a project in which I failed but didn't give up. Can't make projects out of people—another lesson Peter taught me. He was the youngest of seven children and had never had a sibling he could exercise dominion over. That little sibling became me. He teased me mercilessly and encouraged me relentlessly. I'd introduce him to guys I was dating, and Peter always had something to say. He could barely wait till they were out the door: "He's a joker." "You can do better than that." Or his favorite: "For crying out loud, Alua, he's nowhere near as smart as you." He'd groan and roll his eyes and look at me like I'd lost every bit of sense. Then he'd remind me that I should never settle. I'm pretty clear about what he'd say about some of the recent choices I've made in men. In these ways, our dead stay with us.

After a year, Bozoma and Peter were engaged to be married. I was overjoyed. I was going to get to keep him as my big brother *and* I got to be the maid of honor at their wedding. Bridezilla Bozoma insisted that I not loc my hair prior to their wedding because of a designated hairstyle she wanted me to wear. I did it anyway. She was pissed. Her choice in china wasn't my taste and, against my better judgment, I told her one night over the phone when she asked for my opinion. I complained about her to Peter, who laughed it off and reminded me not to get in her way. Here was a man who knew my sister and loved her exactly the way she was. I couldn't have asked for any more from a brother-in-law. For an additional family member I didn't get to choose, I'd hit the jackpot.

When their first daughter, Eve, was born at twenty-three weeks in 2008 and never took a first breath, I got on the first flight to New York from Los Angeles to be with them. Their grief was dense and filled up their small one-bedroom apartment on the Upper East Side. Peter and I would go on long walks so Bozoma could have some time away from his worried and cautious gaze. Welcome or not, I visited often that year. I wanted to keep eyes and hands on my sister as she journeyed through inconceivable pain.

While I usually slept on the couch or air mattress during my visits, sometimes Peter would let me have the bed with her and we'd stay up and talk, or not talk at all. Not being able to fix her pain crushed me, and Peter and I commiserated about it, while also making space for his grief, which he often sidelined in favor of hers. Peter cared deeply about the experiences of others.

Their second daughter, Lael, was born nine weeks premature in 2009, on my birthday. I arrived at the hospital in New York before dawn on a red-eye flight to find Peter bouncing around the lobby waiting for me. I thought I was going to explode; he was like a souped-up Labrador puppy. Downright giddy. "She's here. She's perfect. She's here! And it's your birthday!" he repeated in the elevator to the delivery floor, unable to stand still even though he'd been up all night and it was 6 A.M. Of all the days to be born early, Lael had chosen my special day. Once we reached the room, he left to get a snack and to give Bozoma and me a little time together with our mother. As I walked in, Bozoma said, "You like your birthday gift?" Lael was in the NICU, where she would stay for some time to come. I couldn't wait to see her.

I crawled into the armchair at the foot of the delivery bed with my mom, while my sister was poked and prodded by the nurses. Right away my mom asked me if I needed a nap and what I wanted to eat. I instantly felt thirteen and wanted her to stop fussing over me. Recognizing that exactly thirty-one years prior my mother was in the delivery room giving birth to me, I softened toward her.

When Peter came back from his walk, he had two cupcakes with the numbers 0, for Lael, and 31, for me. We posed for a picture. Bozoma held up the cupcake for Lael, and I held up mine. He smashed my cupcake in my face just as the shutter snapped. I found that photo when combing through his digital pictures searching for an image to use for his funeral program. I cried hot and quiet tears into his computer.

The path to Peter's death was slow at first, then it seemed to happen all at once and amid other family crises. My mother, who'd moved herself to northern New Jersey to help Bozoma and Peter out, was diagnosed with Stage 2 uterine cancer a few months after I'd come back from Cuba. She waited until I was on a trip to South Africa to tell me because she knew I'd cancel my trip to be with her and she wanted me to go and enjoy myself. I was angry with her for not telling me sooner and decided to reroute my return trip to New Jersey for her chemo appointments. After six weeks roaming the South African countryside and falling in love with a German traveler named Patrick—a drummer with brown hair and brown eyes as deep as chocolate swimming pools—I arrived in New Jersey.

My mom and I spent the morning of my thirty-fifth birthday together at the "infusion bar." Quite a sexy name for a toxic medicinal treatment center. This was her second dance with cancer. A few years earlier, she'd been diagnosed with breast cancer, which was treated with a lumpectomy and chemo. My mom tends to be a challenging patient, but she knew the drill—ports, nausea, and pomegranate juice because it *might* help slow the reproduction of cancer cells. The suggestions from friends were endless and frustrating, like drinking

Puerto Rican aloe vera juice instead of doing chemo, and lying on her back with her legs open . . . to let the cancer air out. It was asinine. She is known for her strength, and so the weakness in her body from the treatments rattled me. Despite all the time I spend thinking about death, considering my mother's mortality still unnerves me. It was one of my greatest honors to care for her in ways similar to how she once cared for me, down to fussing over what she ate and asking about her sleep schedule and her bowel movements.

Since I was with my mom, it was the first time I missed Lael's birthday party. Unselfishly, Bozoma and Peter made it a point to include me in all Lael's birthday celebrations. In previous years we'd had matching tutus, accessories, and color schemes—true birthday twins. That year, Lael's fourth and my thirty-fifth, was an afternoon party in a park, with water gun fights and balloons. My sister and Peter promised to bring Lael to my mom's house after the party, so we'd still get to spend some of our special day together.

Bozoma arrived at my mother's house with Lael but without Peter. She told us that he'd fainted in the middle of the party and had gone home to rest. No big deal, he'd said. He was probably dehydrated and coming down with a little something because his throat had been sore for weeks.

That little something turned out to be Stage 4 Burkitt's lymphoma.

Suddenly it felt like a meteor was headed our way. It shattered any veneer that the world is a just place where brothers-in-law, fathers, husbands, sons, friends, people live just because we love them and cannot imagine life without them.

The next four months passed in a prickly flash. I was either in L.A. handling business and quickly repacking my bags, with Patrick traveling around Europe, voraciously reading about death and dying, or visiting my mom and Peter while they were ill in New Jersey and New York. My mom's body was responding to treatment. Peter wasn't faring so well.

I took him to a doctor's appointment one afternoon to check on the Ommaya port they'd put in his head, which would deliver chemo directly to his cerebrospinal fluid. It was giving him intense headaches. "I feel like a cyborg," he said while we waited for the doctor. His head was shaved and I could see the roundish imprint of the device in his skull, along with the stitches where they'd opened his scalp to insert it. It resembled a bite mark. His blue veins drew a map under his thin white scalp, which had never before seen the sun.

"You kinda look like one," I retorted weakly. Then I crossed my eyes, hunched my shoulders, and slurped imaginary drool, like a B-movie zombie. He spat out a giggle while holding his head, then snorted. That made me laugh. Feeding off one another's amusement, we reached a fever pitch. The doctor entered the room to meet our raucous laughter. I laughed so hard I cried that afternoon. I couldn't tell if I was laughing out of joy or out of desperation for joy. It wasn't looking good for Peter. The cancer was spreading faster than they could contain it.

In October of that year, Patrick came to visit me on his first trip to the United States. We drove to Mexico and had a decadent lobster dinner in Rosarito, drinking too many margaritas to drive back to L.A. that night. Continuing our trip north up the Pacific Coast Highway in my Jeep, we stopped in little towns like Cambria to get kettle corn at the farmers market and Pismo Beach to take pictures with the sign. I'm a huge fan of the movie *Clueless*, in which the main character, Cher, becomes the head of the Pismo Beach Disaster Relief Fund, so stopping for that photo was imperative. Our meandering trip up and down the coast was to take three weeks, cresting in the Bay Area. Time together with Patrick came at a premium because we lived on different continents. We wanted to maximize it.

A few days into our trip, we stopped at a restaurant in Big Sur named Nepthene. It's nestled in trees facing the coast and is famous for its epic views of the coastline. It's named after a fictional medicine for chasing away sorrow in Homer's *Odyssey*. It turned out to be a cruel joke. I ordered a glass of rosé and french fries and Patrick ordered a beer—so predictable as a German. He went to the restroom and I turned my phone on to see if there was any cell service. There was none so we enjoyed our drinks and the view, and wandered the grounds for an hour.

As we entered the gift shop, my phone began to buzz in my pocket. When I looked at it, the notifications rolled in like credits after a movie. Bozoma had called three times. My father had called twice and sent a text message asking me to call him as soon as I could. My mother's voice on voicemail sounded desperate. She still used voicemail like an answering machine, as though I could hear her and would pick up the phone. "Okay, Alua. You're not there? Call me as soon as you can, okay?" Aba had called. Ahoba had called. But Peter had called first. It wasn't unlike us to all call each other when there was big news but this was excessive, even for our chatty family.

Puzzled and distressed, I ran back to the car while Patrick paid for his souvenir. My mom was the only one who'd left a voicemail, so I called her back. Plus she'd have the gentlest touch.

Her voice was sweet, not matching the desperation in her voicemail. "So how's your trip, Alua?"

"Hi, Mom. What is it?" I was impatient, instantly regretting her gentle touch.

"Oh, why are you asking?" she said innocently.

"Because you all blew up my phone! Is it you? Is it Peter? Is it Daddy? What's happening?" I couldn't restrain my edginess. Concerned, Patrick approached the car and opened the passenger side door for me. I buckled my seat belt with one hand while I held the phone with the other.

"Well, you know . . . I thought it was important to tell you that . . . well, you know that Peter hasn't been doing so well lately . . . annnnd . . .

well, I thought you should know that . . ." Now her soft touch was killing me. I would have rather had someone serve it to me straight, no salt, no lube, no chaser.

"Mom! What is it??!!" I was panicking.

"And the doctors are saying that they don't know if they can treat his cancer anymore."

The wind in the trees, the traffic on the street, and the air around me became eerily still but for a little piece of dust visible to me in the ray of sunlight in the car. I watched it fall slowly till it fell out of the light. Only then did I become acutely aware of my quickening breath and my heartbeat. Soon Peter wouldn't have either. Using my silence as permission, she continued.

"They can't say how long but they are saying that his time is running short. I know you are on a trip so maybe you should take your time and come when you can."

"No, I'll come immediately." I hung up in a hurry, eager to get on the road and sort through the logistics. Only then did I look up and notice that the car wasn't moving, and Patrick wasn't inside it. Struggling with the seat belt to release me to go find him, my frustration grew. The seat belt doubled down and stiffened across my neck. I yanked at it and yelled, taking out my fear and sadness on this inanimate object just as Patrick appeared and jumped in the driver's seat.

"We have to go. Now!"

"What happened, baby? Are you okay? It seemed serious so I left you alone."

"You left me alone because you thought it was serious? Wouldn't you think I needed you here if it was serious? WHERE WERE YOU??" Uncharacteristically, I screamed at him. My anger typically shows up as sadness first, but in this case, anger led. It was misguided.

I was angry at God, and wondered if there was one at all. I was angry at Burkitt's lymphoma. I was angry at Peter for being sick. I was angry at the seat belt. I was angry at the doctors. I was angry at my mom for delivering the news. I was just angry. Patrick was awestruck, looking at me blankly while taking me in. He'd never heard me yell and rather than react in kind, he waited patiently for me to calm down, sensing that whatever was happening was bigger than him.

"Peter," I whispered, then paused, unsure of how I would say the next words. Once they came out of my mouth, they would be true. I was safer with the words inside. Everyone was safer with the words inside. Perhaps this is why medical teams struggle to say that someone is dying. Once spoken, words are real. Patrick reached for my hand across the center console to bolster me while I found the courage.

"He's dying."

I wept silently until we reached San Francisco, looking out the window at the sky to see if I could actually spot the meteor coming toward my family.

After a sleepless night, Patrick and I wandered around the city and planned our trips out of California—me to New York to see Peter, and Patrick back home to Germany. Despite being raised an evangelical Christian, I'm not a praying gal. My parents still believe, and I think they always will; they've always held out hope for me. I used to be annoyed when they'd ask if I'd gone to church on Sunday, but I also understood the pain they must feel that their daughter might be going to hell for not accepting Jesus Christ as her Lord and Savior. If I had a daughter, I would try to save her from this fate too, I think. Cheekily, I started saying yes when they asked if I'd been to church because, as far as I was concerned, I had. I experience church on hikes. I find the divine in the bees and trees. I have worship at brunch with friends. Or in bed. Laughter is a form of prayer. So is sex.

Nonetheless, I left a desperate prayer that day in the Mission Dolores Basilica for Peter, for my sister, and for Lael. Funny how we turn to a higher power when life feels like it is out of our control.

Patrick and I made it back to L.A. in record time the following day. I packed a small carry-on bag thinking I'd be in New York for just a short while. At my departure gate that night, we shared a tearful and tentative goodbye, unsure of when we'd hug again. Our goodbyes were normally sad because of the distance between us, but this goodbye had a unique and dense quality to it. I fiddled with the buttonhole of his gray cardigan at the airport gate, avoiding teary eye contact while they announced that my flight was boarding. We knew exactly what lay ahead, and still I was choosing to walk into it.

Two months later, I was still in New York. Peter, Bozoma, and Lael's needs kept growing as Peter got sicker. I couldn't leave. I didn't want to. As when Eve was stillborn and grief took hold of them, I slept on the couch at night and researched answers to uncomfortable questions, offered lightness, an ear and comic relief during the day. Sleep was hard to find and offered no escape. I dreamt of getting caught in torrential downpours, swarmed by crows, swallowed by cracks in the earth. Staying asleep was harder than being awake and yet each day greeted us with fresh disastrous news. Peter's potassium levels had dropped drastically one day. His kidneys were failing another. His left eye started roaming in its socket due to a weakened muscle. Medications that were supposed to have one intended outcome caused a number of side effects, which created the need for new medications. Peter was in and out of the hospital, but his spirits were mostly great. On my way on a trip to the drugstore to get a thicker lotion for his drying skin, he cautioned me against getting bottles that were too big. "I won't be needing much of it," he offered with a giggle. The suggestion was unbearable in its stark truth.

We found ways to inject humor and gaiety into an otherwise bleak time. A ceramic toothpick holder from their kitchen, which to me looked like a waiter, became a pill caddy. I'd load up Peter's medicines, carefully following the color-coded timetable posted on the fridge, and present them to him with a deep curtsy and a sip of juice. "Your drugs, my lord." He'd grab the caddy and shoo me away with his nose hilariously turned up. On a trip to Home Depot, in which he insisted on accompanying me, he drove the portable wheelchair cart because he was too weak to stand but wanted a sense of normalcy. I rode on the back pretending we were explorers in a distant and exotic land while looking for boxes to pack up things in the apartment. "Onward . . . AWAAAAYYYYY!" I'd yell. He'd chuckle and respond in a pirate's accent, "Aye, matey!"

Those boxes stayed packed for months after his death.

Peter's elderly parents came to town from Florida and stayed. Thankfully, Bozoma and Peter had moved into a larger apartment on Central Park West in Harlem. His older siblings, who lived in Florida and Massachusetts, also visited during that time. Peter's brother Neil taught me how to make a pecan pie, Peter's favorite, for Thanksgiving, which we held in the hospital along with his other brother, Stephen, their parents, and my mother. His sister, Debbie, and I drank white wine at the kitchen table at night and talked about our shared brother. Ahoba and Aba came to town when they could to help carry the load. Ahoba also had her hands full raising my nephew, Jahcir, while working full-time. My father's visits always came with a lot of prayer, but I never knew what to pray for.

It was an emotionally and physically draining time. To my surprise, I was the most alert, on task, and on fire that I'd ever been. I was supposed to be the aimless one, prone to declaring dozens of short-lived new passions. Sewing, travel photography, jewelry making, UV-cured gel nails, Tae Bo teaching, marathon running. I would travel to one destination, decide to live there, only to bounce to the neighboring country because of a tip from a fellow traveler. My family laughed about my wanderlust. Years later, I made a friend who knew me as an acquaintance during this time. When asked, she said she thought I was an "international floater" before I found death work. And it's no wonder. Death injects purpose into our lives when we let it. I let it rush in. It grounded me, giving a "why" to each day.

Peter was the first person I doula'd before knowing what it was or what I was supposed to be doing. Instinctively, I had found my way to a position that I would go on to assume time and time again. To serve as a death doula is to provide a ring in the circle of support, which radiates outward like the rings in a tree trunk. At the center, Peter journeyed toward his death, supported by my sister and his parents. I occupied the next ring, handling everyone's needs to allow them to focus on what was happening.

Granted, I was also losing my brother, and balancing my grief with that responsibility took effort, but I had my own friends and Patrick, who represented yet another ring of the support circle, to help me when I felt depleted. The shock waves from grief travel far, and constellations of care are wide.

I ran a *lot* of errands during this time, shuttled people back and forth—to the airport, the hospital, home, school, restaurants, and on and on. When the doctors left Peter's hospital room, I'd ask if he and Bozoma understood what was said and made notes for further questions. When my sister took up residence at the hospital after Peter was admitted for the last time, I packed a bag for her and bought pajamas that she could throw away when this was over. She'd never want to see them again. I also snuck sparkling Shiraz into the hospital and sat in the family room with her most nights. These moments away created space for her to talk about the things she couldn't talk about in front of Peter—her exhaustion, her fear, her questions. We bought notecards for Peter to write letters to Lael to open when she was older. That chance never came, as he quickly became too weak to hold a pen. With Bozoma at Peter's bedside, the majority of their daughter Lael's care was left to me, her Aunty Mommy.

It was a busy time. I'd take Lael to school in the morning and after she finished for the day, I'd pick her up in Harlem and drive her to midtown to the hospital to spend a few hours with her parents and do her four-year-old's "homework." After she'd get restless in the little hospital room with all the machines, buttons, beeps, and lights, we'd say good night, and I'd take her home for dinner and get her ready for bed. Some nights we'd make crafts for her parents. After

Lael fell asleep, a friend of Bozoma's would come for the night so I could head back to the hospital to check in on everyone.

When I was exhausted or Peter's condition seemed particularly precarious, I'd sometimes spend the night in a chair in his hospital room. In the mornings, I'd wake before Lael did, drive home, and get her ready for school. Those last few weeks of Peter's life were one long treacherous day of power naps, looking for parking in New York City, snacks instead of meals, doctors, misinformation, hospital elevator banks, and impending doom.

Lael and I, already close, had a lot of intimate time during those months. Little kids are particularly inquisitive about death. Not only are they in the "why" asking phase of development, but according to Swiss developmental psychologist Jean Piaget, at four years old they are starting to grapple with the notion of object impermanence. Can things/people go away forever? Lael's questions on sleepy Saturday mornings before we made pancakes and I plopped her down in front of cartoons did not disappoint. "Where do we go when we die?" After asking her what she thought, I'd ask her what her mother said. It was important to keep the message consistent, and I knew better than to interfere in big conversations between a parent and a child who wasn't mine. I'm deferring to her mom as Lael grows and continues to ask me tough questions—like why people groom their pubic hair. She's always been inquisitive, and she gets that trait from me, her fellow Gemini.

Lael asked if Peter's ears would grow very large. Someone had told her that her dad would be able to hear her from heaven after he died, and since she couldn't visit heaven, she sensed it was far away. She asked if Peter would go back to where he was before he was born, the place she had recently come from. Children know a lot more about death than we think. Her questions were tough, and it pained me to tell her that I didn't know the answers while also providing safety and comfort to her. She asked if I was going to die too. I told her that

I planned to be around for a long time. When we avoid children's questions about death, we inadvertently communicate that they should shove their scary thoughts down. That ultimately reinforces a death-phobic culture. Talking to children about death is a delicate balance, but I believe we owe them the truth of our "I don't know, but what I do know is. . . " I wish I knew more of the answers for Lael's sake. And for mine too, especially when the reality of Peter's impending death was approaching. We were woefully unprepared.

Generally, I remember wishing we had a lot more information. It would have been invaluable to ask someone about how to talk to children about death. Or how I should approach the topic of Peter's burial or cremation decisions. Or what the signs of dying were. Or just to have someone to say, "This is normal. You guys are doing great. This fucking sucks. I've got you," would have been worth its weight in gold. These statements are in my doula bag now, and I dole them out like Halloween candy when working with families, depending on their level of offense at my sailor's mouth. I would have paid my weight in gold for someone to remind us to be intentional in our actions in the last few days of Peter's life and to offer ways to say goodbye with grace.

I also wish someone had explained the death rally to us. Sometimes called "terminal lucidity," this is the period in which a dying person appears more alert, stable, and energized. They start making plans, cracking jokes, and reminiscing with their families. After days of refusing food, they might ask for a meal. It can resemble a turnaround in the health of the dying beloved, but it is the opposite. People seeing this for the first time think they're witnessing the miracle they have been hoping for. What they're actually witnessing is a standard, normal sign that death is near. Flowers smell the most beautiful just before they wither; so too does the death rally flare with that last little bit of life's fire before it dies.

On Sunday, December 8, 2013, Peter rallied. The New England Patriots were playing the Cleveland Browns. Peter was a huge Patriots fan, but at this point he was also a husk of himself—emaciated, depressed, and lethargic. He had barely spoken in days. That's why I was surprised and delighted to hear his voice on the other end of my cell phone, asking me to bring Lael to the hospital in her tiny Patriots jersey.

I also wanted to yell "booooo" into the phone. My sisters and I were Broncos fans, and Peter knew this. Shit-talking the Patriots to him was one of my favorite pastimes. But he was dying. The least I could do was let him cheer on his team in peace, right? And boy, did he know it. He milked it. The fucking Patriots. I wondered if this level of self-sacrifice would get me nominated for the Nobel Peace Prize. For a second, I also thought about sneaking Lael's Broncos jersey under the other one, although after some deliberation, I realized that doing so would make her too hot. (But yes, I am that petty.)

Lael and I showed up at the hospital to find Peter sitting up in bed. He still looked like he was dying, but doing so in the middle of a tailgate, cracking jokes and giving orders to his friends and family, including Bozoma, my mother, and his parents, who were still in town. Where had the man of the past few weeks gone? Peter felt like the old Peter again, although he was also impossibly thin, immobile, totally bald, and verbally challenged because of the tumors growing on his vocal cords. It was hard for me to reconcile that this sick version of Peter was also Peter. He asked his best friend, Mecca, to get a park bench in Central Park dedicated to him after his death. He whispered private requests to others. I took notes. The blossoming death doula in me was hard at work making sure his wishes were noted. At one point, I heard Peter ask for whiskey, as though we were at a sports bar and not the bedside of a frail, ill, and weak man. Quizzically, I looked at Bozoma. She shrugged.

What the hell is going on?

Before the game was over, Peter's rally ran out of gas and he asked for some quiet time. One by one, his friends said something to the effect of "See you later, brother" and left. As Lael's bedtime drew near, it was time for me to take her home to get her ready for school the next day. Since it seemed he was doing pretty well, I spent the night at home to give Peter, Bozoma, and his mom and dad some space. The chairs in his hospital room were prime real estate and one less person meant that someone else could put their feet up on my chair to sleep.

Unaware that it would be the last time I said goodbye to Peter, I was nonchalant when he told me he was tired. He'd been so vibrant that day. So much like his old self and unlike someone who was close to death, despite all the signs. I hoped that this was our miracle, but my gut was cautious. After we said good night, I went home with Lael, put her to sleep, and poured myself a glass of wine. Patrick was the first person I called, and I asked him to tell me about his day to restore some normalcy to our relationship. Then I called my dad, Ahoba, and Aba to give updates. They'd all visited at various points throughout Peter's illness, but couldn't uproot themselves for the long haul like I did. Being the wanderer in the family, it turns out, has some advantages. Utterly exhausted after the calls, I fell asleep on the couch with half a glass of wine in my hand (the rest spilled on my pants), and woke up with a stiff neck just in time to greet the sun.

I dropped Lael off at school and went to print family photos for one of her class projects. When I reached the hospital room that morning after picking up eye drops for Peter's father, the mood was somber. My mom sat in the crevice between Peter's room and the one next to it on the phone. Eyes swollen and hair disheveled, Bozoma sat on Peter's right side clutching his arm. His mother was on his left with a fixed gaze on Peter's hand. His father absently looked out the window at nothing in particular. Although it was past 10 A.M., Peter hadn't yet woken. He would never wake up again.

For three days and nights we sat vigil by his bedside as Peter labored out of this world. Christmas, two weeks away, was his favorite holiday. We played Christmas songs and wore Santa hats. A nurse with a serious set of pipes came to sing a few Christmas carols for him. Palliative care doctors floated in cautiously to check on him. There was apology in their movements and voices, without uttering one. It was clear what was happening, yet no one dared to say the words to name this confusing, liminal state. Peter was actively dying.

Sometime around 3 A.M. on Wednesday, December 11, 2013, I felt a stirring in the hospital room. I woke up to find Peter's mother nudging his father awake. Bozoma was already awake with her eyes fixated on Peter's chest, observing his irregular breathing pattern of deep breaths, followed by shallow ones. We rejoiced whenever he took another labored breath through his mouth, which lay open for days, though I don't know what we were rejoicing for. Another breath meant he was still alive. But it also meant he was still suffering. And it meant that his death process would be longer. But no more breaths meant Peter was gone. Both equally devastating, and neither offering relief. Pure, exacting agony in a breath.

Bozoma held her position at his right side with his mother on his left. Peter's father touched his left leg while holding hands with his wife, watching their last-born son die. My mom stood behind Bozoma with her hands on her shoulders. As I'd done countless times before, I took my position at Peter's feet, which I'd regularly massaged with moisture-rich lotion to prevent them from cracking. Today, they were cold and yellowing, due to jaundice. I've since learned that in some faith traditions, the soul disengages from the feet first to leave through the head. I held them, quietly and tearfully thanking him for walking the earth and walking into my life, and wished him well for wherever he was walking to next.

Shortly before 4 A.M., four days before his forty-fourth birthday, my brother-in-love Peter Saint John breathed his last.

The room filled with a deafening stillness until Bozoma pierced it with a sharp and defeated whimper. Her husband and father of her children, Eve and Lael, was dead. From one breath to the next, the spark of life left Peter's body. He would make no new memories. He would say no more words. He would never touch us again. We would never hear his voice again. His big body, which had housed an entire human life and the depth of our love, returned to the very matter it was made of. It would soon disintegrate in fire when he was cremated. Ashes to ashes. Peter would be gone, but the gift of his life will remain in every life he touched and all the lives we touch, for we carry him with us.

Four days later, on a heavily snowy Sunday, we held his funeral at a Catholic cathedral. Afterward, we threw him a forty-fourth birthday party. There were party hats, balloons, whiskey, and cigars. I looked for him in every nook of the restaurant, knowing he wouldn't appear. But I couldn't help myself. He would have loved the party. He should have been there. But he wasn't. The permanence of his death hadn't landed in my bones and still evades me many years later. I still can't believe he isn't here, hasn't seen Lael as a teenager, hasn't seen me as old as he was when he died, hasn't seen what we created from his death. I still look for him.

He came to me, just once, in a grief dream.

In this dream I've stumbled upon a big street parade. Similar to Mardi Gras in New Orleans, with people of all races, shapes, sizes, and ages wearing many colors, hats, costumes, and jewelry, dancing around each other. They are vibrant in their festival best, worn like everyday clothing. A far-off gentle drum like a heartbeat heard on an ultrasound provides the soundtrack. Glitter floats in the air as far as I can see. I am in awe of this enchanted place, where people live in bold color and breathe glitter rather than oxygen, but I approach the crowd cautiously. I am an outsider, and everyone else inhabits the space like they belong.

Off to the right, I see a large float in the shape of a goldfish dec-

orated in tennis ball–sized cobalt-blue and lime-green sequins. The
shiny deep green back fin of the fish waves effortlessly side to side,
giving the impression that the giant fish is swimming down the
street in glitter water. Standing alone at the top of the fish's fluores-
cent yellow fin like a captain is my beloved Peter in his full regality.
I am relieved to see someone familiar but shocked by his outfit. He's
wearing a purple and turquoise sparkly top hat, a bright turquoise
satin tie with no shirt, and fuchsia latex pants with silver platform
boots. I'm equally embarrassed that he's out here shirtless and tickled
that he's so free. Minus the costume, he looks like a version of himself who wasn't sick. Tall, vital, robust, with both eyes facing forward,
not one roaming because of a wonky muscle.

Peter spots me in the crowd, and excitedly makes his way down
the float and through the crowd to me. I jump to hug him and weep
in joy to lay my dream eyes on him. Peter laughs at my tears. I think
people here probably don't cry, except in bliss. He asks me how I got
here and I tell him I don't know. I just arrived. I don't belong but
this place is full of color and rapturous love, and I want to stay. It
reminds me of Burning Man. I always wanted to go there with him.
Peter affirms that I am not supposed to be here, but jokes that he's
not at all surprised that I've broken the rules. We laugh again, and it's
refreshing to be with him in this way. Peter knows me as a disruptor
and he's not wrong, even in the dream world.

I try to ask questions about where we are. But he won't answer
and gets worried that someone will see me and starts looking around
anxiously. I look around too, but all I see is jubilation. Not an ounce
of threat.

The longer Peter stands with me, the more anxious he becomes.
Eventually he tells me that he has to hop back on his big psychedelic
fish, which is swimming along without him. I beg him to stay but I
am torn because he was so happy on the float and instead, he is now
worried about me. I don't want him to be worried, but the thought
of being separated from him again is unbearable. I've experienced

the acute pain of grief from his death once, and I don't want to do it again. Now that he is with me, he *must must must* stay. The party is moving on behind him and I am bereft that he is leaving. I beg and plead with him and then see that it pains him also to leave me. But he must. So I relent, defeated. While everything inside of me is screaming for my brother-in-love to stay with me just a little longer, not to leave me here without him, I will let him go because it is best. He belongs here.

Peter takes off his top hat and streaks of colorful light shoot off his head. His Ommaya is still visible but his dirty-blond hair has grown back around it, brushing his ears. He needs a haircut. And a damn shirt. He places the hat on my head and I grab ahold of it with both hands, pushing it down on my head and feeling the bits of glitter that are stuck to it. He asks me if I feel the glitter with my fingers. I nod yes. I can feel the crinkly texture and sharp edges. He asks me if I see the glitter on my fingers and in the air. I say yes—little dancing flecks of shiny purple and turquoise in my vision field and on my hands. Peter looks at me soberly, in stark contrast to the excitement around us. He tells me that I was only supposed to come with him to the gate, that I shouldn't have followed him inside like a tagalong little sister. I must turn around. He is loving. Kind. And firm. Like the big brother he was to me in life.

With those words and no goodbye, Peter turns around and runs off into the crowd in his silver boots to chase his shiny floating fish. He doesn't look back at me. I start to back away, wanting to hold on to this euphoric place, until the entire scene is full of only glittery sparkles. The colorful people are gone. The party is gone. His float is gone. Peter is gone.

I wake up from this dream in Patrick's home, in dark and damp Berlin, with wet, puffy eyes. I am sad about how real it felt because I cannot feel it anymore. He might be off on a psychedelic fish adventure in the dream world, but in the default physical world, Peter is still dead. And we must go on without him.

A week or so after Peter's funeral, I couldn't focus on any tasks. And there was so much to do. Maybe it was the grief, or maybe it was the utter lack of boundaries and self-care that depleted me. Patrick had repeatedly asked me to come to Germany to be with him. I would swear to him that everything was okay, but my sweet boyfriend encouraged me to let him take care of me for a while. After a few days of insisting that I was fine but not being able to remember how to put pants on (*Do you sit down to do it? Does the button go first or the zipper? Fuck it, I'll wear a skirt*), I agreed with him. Maybe it was the grief, maybe it was the exhaustion. Thinking about leaving Bozoma alone for the first time in months crushed me, but I was no longer any good to her because I was no good to myself. I was spent and empty. Self-care must be a priority as we usher others toward death. I didn't know that yet.

Using a pad of brightly colored sticky notes, I sat at the dining room table one afternoon, attempting to quickly outline the tasks that needed to get done so that we could wrap up Peter's affairs before I left for Germany. I thought I would only use a couple. But one small task quickly ballooned to thirty.

Contact credit card companies and reporting agencies.

Catalogue and close online bills and accounts.

Get access to Peter's email account.

Figure out what to do with his clothes. Clean his closet now or hold off?

Return medical equipment.

Sort through his mail.

Contact the Social Security Administration.

Locate his birth certificate and insurance policies.

Determine if Peter is subject to probate [the process through which courts legally decide who inherits what, after someone has died].

Find the title to his car.

This last sticky I remember vividly because of the maze of paper-work it triggered. Peter wanted to gift his car—a maroon Mitsubishi Eclipse—to his nephew. I thought all we had to do was give the nephew the keys. So foolish of me to think it would be that simple, or that the rules in place for transferring a car title after a loved one's death would favor the grieving. No, no—the process of transferring a title to a vehicle after a death when it hasn't been properly trans-ferred in any testamentary document, like a last will and testament or a trust, *is a nightmare* that even non-grieving people don't want to carry out. Who wants to sit at the DMV on a regular day, let alone in the midst of deep grief?

There were so, so many instances like this. I'd call a credit card company to tell them that Peter had died, only for them to ask to speak to him to get verification that I was authorized to handle his account. *He's DEAD, asshole.* Every time that I had to repeat that he was dead, I fell deeper into the grief pit. And simultaneously the death duties mounted. If I, the valiant juris Doctor–carrying sister-in-law, couldn't make sense of the myriad things to do to wrap up my brother-in-law's affairs, how could my heavily grieving sister? How could people who don't have any support at all? The sticky notes filled too quickly. I was a whole pad of little four-by-four-inch sticky notes in, and hadn't scratched the surface. I looked at Bozoma sitting on the couch, in pajamas at 4 P.M., her hair still tied back in a scarf, staring into nothingness—while the TV, on the same channel for the past six hours, blared nonsense to drown the emptiness.

At that moment I would have offered a kidney on the black market for someone to help us. Why wasn't there someone thoughtful, com-passionate, knowledgeable, and kind to help? Someone who could explain the order in which to close out Peter's accounts? That took me at least twelve sticky notes. Or suggestions for what to do with the hospital equipment at home? Six sticky notes. What on earth were we supposed to do with all the leftover medications? Four. Where would I find out which insurance policies he had? Fourteen.

The dining room table was littered in yellow, green, orange, and pink notes that held no answers. Just more questions leading a trail that circled back to the same place. Peter was dead and we didn't have the information we needed to wrap up his affairs. It had died with him.

Intellectually, I understood that there were hundreds of thousands of people who were struggling with similar tasks. According to the Medindia medical review's World Population Clock, over 150,000 people across the world die each day. To some extent, all of them have lives that need closing out after their deaths. Peter was not the first person to die nor would he be the last. Then why did the experience of his death feel so isolating? Why did I feel so alone as I tried to help? And what the fuck kind of society understands the universality of a painful experience but does next to nothing about it? Why do we leave each other alone in our pain? It was like being with Jessica on that bus in Cuba all over again, knowing for sure that she wasn't the only one who had thoughts about dying, but that she'd been left alone in it. Except this time it was happening in my family.

Heaven help the social worker who told me to do an internet search to figure out the probate process. I cursed their children's children and they caught *all* of my anger (read: grief). The hospital suggested that the funeral home could help. The funeral home told me they would call Social Security on our behalf, but that we were on our own with sorting out Peter's other business. They suggested that I reach out to hospice.

I thought hospice was only a place where people went to die. I was wrong. Hospice is a theory of care, not a place, which shifts the focus from curative to qualitative care, with a specialized team of folks to support that care. People can receive hospice services anywhere. But the medical care team at Peter's hospital stopped trying to cure him too late so he never got a referral before he died. It felt like he was cheated. The hospice told me that their bereavement services might help with my frustration (read: grief), but that they had no services to help with the bureaucracies I kept finding myself up against. Where were the people who were supposed to help in times like this? We have professionals who guide us through every step of our lives otherwise. Tutors help with schoolwork when we aren't learning efficiently. Wedding planners help plan weddings. Real estate agents help sell houses. Counselors help navigate relationships. Birth doulas support people through the birthing process. Hell, there are even professional snugglers. So why aren't there people to help when it comes to the end of a life?

My desire to cure societal ills often fuels my actions. It led me to become a vegetarian as a kid and to enter the professional workforce as a Legal Aid attorney making forty thousand dollars per year, while my law school buddies went corporate and made hundreds of thousands of dollars. My entry into death work was no different. For me, death work is activism at its core. Fueled by anger but cloaked in love.

Most of us who come to the practice of death work come from a similar place. Either we witnessed a death so beautiful and idyllic that we want everyone to experience the same, or we sat by and watched a loved one suffer while suffering ourselves and we never want another to bear the same burden. In both cases, we come to improve the experience for others. I came to death work because I wanted to help "fix" the system I saw.

I wanted to throw a Molotov cocktail at the entire healthcare/deathcare (or lack thereof) apparatus.

I didn't want anyone else to suffer the way that my family had.

I wanted someone to speak clearly to us that Peter was dying.

I wanted someone to explain the signs of dying.

I wanted the palliative care team to speak their apologies rather than just wear it on their shoulders.

I wanted someone to be there to help sort the bureaucratic mess.

I wanted to make Peter's death as ideal as it could be, given the fucked-up, my-big-brother-is-dying-from-an-aggressive-cancer-and-

I-can't-help-him circumstances. The death of a loved one sucks for everyone. But what can we do to make it gentler? Just like a child calls attention to an ouchie, we also want to know someone cares that we are hurting.

My displaced anger at sticky notes continues to this day, you should know. But my anger for my sister and for thousands of people caught in the bureaucratic cyclone after a death turned into fuel. If there wasn't anyone I could call to help me, sure as shit I could be the someone others turned to when their loved ones needed them most. I could remind them that they were doing it right. I could sit at the DMV for them. I could learn about the death rally and explain it to them. I could help them figure out how to talk to their children about death. I could empower them to care for their beloveds themselves. I could be *with* them in the trenches. I could hold their hands. I could hold their hearts. And while I couldn't take their pain away, I could let them know that someone cared that it was hard. I could be their witness. I wanted to be.

Chapter 5

Show Up and Shut Up

When I was twelve years old, my dad shook me awake by the shoulder one morning at 4 A.M. "Alu! Aluuuuu. Do you want to come with me?"

I opened my eyes. I didn't know where he was going, but my answer was *always* yes. My father traveled a lot for missionary work, and when he was home, he split his time among me, my three sisters, and my mother. Alone time with him was rare, and when he was gone, I missed him so much that I would smell his clothes. He loved little adventures, and my preteen heart couldn't turn one down—still can't today. Not ever a morning person, I jumped at the opportunity for a mystery mission and got myself dressed.

It was 1990, and we'd been living in Colorado Springs for a year. My dad and I bundled up against the December weather and climbed into our maroon Chrysler station wagon. I removed my fingers from the thick black-and-white glove that matched my hat, to make sure the seat belt snapped into the passenger side seat belt holder. It stuck a little. Touching the cold metal of the seat belt clasp made my fingers numb. I blew hot breath on them, stuffed them back inside the warmth of the glove, and sat on my hands. With the radio on a news channel, my father headed toward the highway. My mother was out of town for a few weeks, and while she had made enough meals to get us through, my dad decided he wanted fresh meat to supplement the meals. My dad is serious about his meat. The sky started to lighten as we set off on our adventure. I was giddy.

An hour and a half later, he pulled off the road somewhere in rural Denver and parked along a fence with a home in the distance. Animals roamed, separated by species. A man greeted us as we got out of the car and he and my father exchanged pleasantries. I spotted goats, cows, and a lot of farm equipment. The smell of manure hung in the air. Finally, we arrived at the chicken coop, where they were already singing cock-a-doodle-doo to greet the day.

Breathing into my scarf to generate heat and to diffuse the pungent smell, I watched the sun rising over the Colorado Rocky Mountains. Then, in the distance, a nightmarish bleating. It was so desperate that I could feel the fear and sadness in my own body. Adrenaline streaked through my chest and into my fingertips, zapping warmth into them. I couldn't breathe. I scrambled to see where the noise was coming from and if I could help, but as in a real nightmare, I couldn't. While my dad surveyed the chickens to select a few, I grew increasingly distraught. Where was the noise coming from? Why was the animal so scared? What was happening to it?

A loud blast sounded, and the bleating came to a sudden halt. It felt as though the shot hit me directly. I instantly burst into tears.

My dad rushed to my side. "What's wrong, Alua? Eh? Why are you crying? What's the problem?"

I couldn't find the words for the shock.

My father's alarm grew and he shook me gently.

"The goat, Daddy," I managed, choking through my tears. "I think they killed a goat."

My dad's eyes narrowed, then quickly widened. He's never handled the tears or discomfort of his daughters well. He's the type of man who laughs so hard he coughs, but as of that morning, I hadn't yet seen him cry. My father always hoped to protect us from pain, and his jovial nature and solid dose of African masculinity didn't leave room for maudlin emotions or big displays. Given that I was full of both, I was a handful.

My runaway passions delighted, flustered, or annoyed my parents, depending on the day. In Colorado Springs, I wanted to paint my basement bedroom bright yellow and to my surprise, they agreed. By the third trip to the paint shop so I could get the paint color *juuuuussst* right, they grew understandably frustrated, but took me anyway. Once when I was a little girl I brought a bug I'd caught into the kitchen, thinking my parents would be equally amazed by the little creature's iridescence. "Take it back outside or I'll kill it!" my mom yelled. Animals and bugs did not belong in the house, and I had enthusiastically trampled a boundary yet again.

That morning at the farm, my father muttered a bunch of words that I couldn't decipher, patted me on the back as though to dislodge something stuck in my throat, and rushed me quickly to the car. He was embarrassed; I was inconsolable. Despite all the danger and risks that my family endured fleeing Ghana, this goat was the closest I'd come to facing a living being's death. How was it crying one minute, breathing one minute, and dead the next? And why had nobody seemed to care but me?

On the ride home from the animal murder horror house, my father tried to explain that this was the way humans got their meat. He'd grown up in a part of Ghana where families are responsible for killing the animals they eat, so this process wasn't unusual to him or most people around the world. Me? I just stared blankly out the car window. I couldn't get my head around it; I'd heard the animal *cry*. I'd felt its pain. How could I ever put animal flesh in my mouth again when I could feel the animal's emotions? The animal was in fear when it died and now I was supposed to *eat* that fear? No way. While I couldn't do much about that one goat, I could choose not to harm another goat.

By the time we arrived home, I was clear that I wouldn't eat any kind of meat again. My father knew better than to keep arguing with his hardheaded and softhearted daughter. So he offered to take me to the only health food store in town at the time to find meat substitutes. And because my father's love also shows up as solidarity, he decided to become a vegetarian with me.

He lasted until lunch.

Back then, the meat substitutes tasted like cardboard. Vegetarianism was still twenty years off from becoming sexy. After gagging through a veggie burger, Dad asked if he could stop being a vegetarian. I laughed and let him off the hook, just grateful he cared.

The goat was an early taste of my own runaway empathy. Empathy feels virtuous, but just like any intense emotional experience, it can be a sort of addiction. It has been for me. My broken heart has served as my north star as far back as I can remember. At age eleven, I fell hard when I learned the story of a teenage boy named Ryan White. By the time my family moved to America from Ghana, Ryan White was already a household name. He was a white child with hemophilia who had contracted the HIV/AIDS virus from a blood transfusion. HIV/AIDS was poorly understood at the time, and teachers, parents, and school administrators were terrified to let Ryan be in class with other kids. Ryan fought back legally and, in doing so, became one of the first people to bring national attention to the AIDS epidemic. His youth and wholesomeness cut against the perception that HIV/AIDS only happened to Black folks, gay men, drug addicts, or bad people—in other words, people who "deserved it."

I became preoccupied with Ryan's ostracism from school and society because of his illness. I couldn't understand why he couldn't go to school like I did because of something his body did. As I learned more through news stories, I ached for the deaths of untold others, who often suffered alone and without family. I was too young to understand the demonization of gay men or the sexuality judgments persistent in how we talked about the illness. But I was sensitive enough to know something was fucked up. It broke my budding-death-doula heart. I sobbed through Ryan's television funeral in 1990, glued to the TV.

Just as it would with the goat a year later, my heartbreak sparked righteousness, which eventually flared into activism. In 2000, the year I graduated from Wesleyan University, I spent the summer in Chiang Mai, Thailand, working in HIV/AIDS education at the YMCA. I held classes on sexual health while my Thai counterparts gathered around me with their fingers in my hair, joking that if a spider got caught in my teeny-weeny Afro, it would get stuck and die. Even though I'd lived twenty-one years with a 4C curl pattern, I washed my hair too often after that day, for fear of it turning into a spider grave site.

That was an enlightening trip, in more ways than one. I learned the importance of understanding a culture's mores and values before discussing topics that are taboo, like death. Or sex. During a weekend trip to Myanmar to expand the reach of the sex ed program, my friends and I showed up at the location where we intended to teach, coordinated by another aid organization, only to find armed guards outside forbidding our entrance. I quickly learned to follow the lead of the community members before asserting myself and my own beliefs. I learned that sometimes ignorance just means lack of access to knowledge and information.

Despite the cultural challenges, I felt more myself in Thailand than I'd ever felt. I had been to other countries before, but now I was older and on my own, with no parents to protect me and no sisters with which to conspire. I was doing work that felt good in my spirit, going on adventures with fellow travelers to the Thai islands, seeing how other humans did life, and eating fresh mangos daily. I couldn't get myself to leave.

I was supposed to fly home from Thailand and start law school, but I delayed my ticket back to the States until I'd missed registration at almost all of the schools I'd gotten into. My dad promised to come get me himself if I pushed my flight back again. I got on the next flight and showed up to register at University of Colorado Boulder School of Law, the last school that would still take me, even though I was late. Walking through the law library stacks, jet-lagged and pissy, I could still smell phantom pad see ew and hear tuk-tuks.

After my first year of law school, I worked at South Brooklyn Legal Services in the HIV/AIDS Unit, pairing my formal education with my youthful Ryan White heartbreak. Finally, I could *do* something tangible about the injustices that broke me in the world.

One of my first clients was Natasha, a slim Black twenty-six-year-old woman with a sunflower tattoo on her neck. Born and raised in Brooklyn, Tash had been formally educated at an elite, competitive college—one of the "Little Ivies"—like the one I'd gone to. She had a short natural haircut like mine and loved to toss big vocabulary in with slang. We'd flip effortlessly among topics like Mary J. Blige, Mumia Abu-Jamal, and Buddhism. She was just as tall as I was, and she had a gap in her front teeth too, albeit a smaller one than mine. Because she had never tried to close it despite suggestions from numerous dentists, I accepted her as a member of the gap-toothed crew. Many of us had to fight to keep our gaps. Tash and I seemed to have so much in common. But Tash had contracted HIV from an old boyfriend. Now she had AIDS, was raising their kid as a single mom, and was on government benefits. All while facing eviction.

Once again, my empathy got the best of me. Her situation felt personal. Day in and day out, I catered to Natasha's needs, far beyond what was required of me as a law student attending to her housing discrimination case. I helped her pick up prescriptions and order meals, and I taught her son how to tie his shoes. I was often tired at work, spending evenings talking to Tash when she was scared, lonely, or needed an errand run.

None of these were part of my job. And yet I felt more alive and more certain of the value I was offering when running these errands then when I was typing out responses to a demand letter. In legal services, I was discovering, there were few opportunities to feel like I was truly helping. No matter how hard we worked, it often felt like sweeping sand on the beach. The system of oppression kept dumping more sand on us. The work was low on immediate gratification.

Tash may have been taking advantage of my generosity, but I didn't care. The relief I sensed she felt when I was near was true—and real—enough for me. Unfortunately, my own needs were going unmet to meet Tash's. This is the danger of those with runaway empathy. Forget just giving you the shirt off our backs. We would give our skin if we could.

Maybe I was enacting some confused version of what my parents instilled in me. They'd spent their lives in service, after all—to the gospel, to family, to community, to us. I might not have ever shared their religious fervor, but maybe some Jesus had snuck into my worldview anyway—*love thy neighbor as thyself*. I seemed to be remembering the first three words and forgetting the last two. It felt holy.

Nearing the end of my summer internship, my supervisor, Cynthia Schneider, called me into her office. I thought I'd be commended on what a good job I was doing with Natasha. Instead, Cynthia told me to back off, in an uncharacteristically blunt manner. When she asked why I was logging so many hours with Tash, my only response was "If it were me, I'd want help doing all of these things too."

Cynthia shook her head somberly. "Well, Alua, it's not you." We sat in silence for a beat while I tried to understand this revolutionary concept. Tash was Black. About my age. Same education. Similar background. An equal. A peer. A sister. And still, she was not me. I could not understand the depth of her experience because I wasn't having it. *What a novel concept.* I'd collapsed the space between myself and Natasha, compounding our experiences and needs. Empathy on crack. I'd also never asked what Tash needed beyond our initial interview and original client retainer. Kindly, Cynthia warned me of burnout and malpractice if I didn't refocus my mind on Tash's legal needs. "Protect your heart," she suggested.

This was perhaps the greatest piece of professional advice I ever received, even trumping the advice to get a CPA when I began Going with Grace, my death doula business. It's important not to conflate others' experience with your own, because then we give them what *we* would want for ourselves rather than what *they* need. That is a common mistake. It's one I've had to learn not to make.

Cynthia's words have carried me through death work, and they come up time and time again. Empathic people often fall repeatedly into this trap. We try to place ourselves in another's shoes. But it simply doesn't work with people who know they are dying, nor with people who are grieving a death. There is no way to put ourselves in their shoes, even if we have had a similar experience.

Part of our desire to put ourselves in another's shoes is to fix the perceived pain of the other. But there is no fixing the pain of grief or death. This means that we must get comfortable with that part of ourselves that feels helpless in the face of another's pain. It might mean long silences. It might mean they don't want your company or your tuna fish casserole. Our support must show up in different ways.

My motto to support the grieving or the dying is simple: show up and shut up. After acknowledging that the situation sucks and you don't know what to say, let them lead the way. If they are silent, be silent with them. If they want to talk about something benign, follow them there. And if they want to talk about their pain, let them talk about *their* pain—not your experience, unless you are asked for it. Just be in the trenches with them and give the incredible gift of bearing witness.

For years I wondered what happened to Natasha. If I had to do it all over again, I probably still would have taught her son how to tie his shoes, but I would have asked her what kind of support she needed and wanted instead of stepping in and trying to be all things to her. I imagine that not long after our work together, Tash died, a victim to an insidious disease. I remain grateful that she taught me the difference between compassion and empathy.

Empathy says: "I know what you are going through." Compassion says: "I might not understand exactly what you are going through, but I am curious about your experience, understand that it is tough, and I am right here with you." I believe compassion is the most healing force on the planet, especially as someone lays dying. Death doulas and those who sit bedside must come from a place of compassion to be effective. From any other place, it is patronizing or paternalistic. Even though well-meaning, it is the equivalent of shoving our love down their throats. For example, have you ever tried to love a friend into sobriety? Or to cajole them to break up with somebody? Ever attempted to convince a loved one to lose a few pounds because you *know* how good it will be for them?

Doesn't work out so well, does it?

The same thing applies in death work. In supporting a client through the dying process, "I know what is better for you than you do" might as well be a cardinal sin. It shows a lack of trust and respect in a client's ability to govern their own lives—and deaths.

So what happens when it seems like the most loving thing to do is to "help someone" accept the fact that they will die? Or to accept the fact yourself that someone you love is dying?

About three-quarters of the calls I get are from well-meaning family members who want me to help their beloved accept the fact that they will die. It's a really terrible position for me to be in: the sick family member thinks I'm the angel of death coming for them. I feel like a jerk and the beloved feels betrayed. No one wins.

Learning to sit alongside our mortality is one of the most important journeys we will take. And it's so personal. We approach death like we approach life. Some people effortlessly hold the truth close, while others hold it at arm's length. Neither is better than the other. Everyone moves in their own time. If we can't convince our best friends to leave their toxic and unsupportive partner, what makes us think that we can force recognition of the deepest existential dilemma on an unwilling human?

Years after I tried and failed to become Tash's personal savior, I came up against this question as a death doula when I meet Akua. Standing at the threshold of her home, I knock gingerly at first, then louder. I can hear what sounds like live music coming from inside, even with the windows closed. While the time of my arrival has been coordinated with her son Reggie, I never quite know in what state I will find my clients. I am certainly not expecting a concert.

A professional caregiver answers the door after a few knocks and lets me into Akua's first-floor apartment. Speakers blare music from every corner and instantly, I recognize Fela Kuti's saxophone and multilayered rhythms. There is barely any space on the red walls, which are covered in African art—masks, paintings, renditions of village life and abstract human figures. The caregiver walks me through the maze of books, wood carvings, and sculptures on the floor on the way to the bedroom. I find Akua in the bed, jovial, slight in stature with a bald head, dancing elegantly with just her skinny arms. This seems highly unusual for someone with the disease progression Reggie mentioned. Could this be her death rally?

"Come in, come in! What an honor it is to receive you in my home!" Akua shouts over the music even with a weakened diaphragm. She draws out her vowels as though she is singing the words. I shout gratitude back as Akua motions to the caregiver to turn down the music. We all approach death in different ways and at this moment, Akua's death is sounding like a rager. I am both bemused and suspicious. What kind of death will this be? What will it require of me?

Born as Helena but coming of age in the sixties, Akua has adopted the Ghanaian name meaning "girl born on Wednesday" for most of her adult life. In her illness, she's reverted to Helena, as she'd never changed her name legally and got tired of correcting doctors. I agree to call her Akua and we marvel over the odds of an African American who has traveled extensively around West Africa finding a Ghanaian death doula in Los Angeles. She tells me she believes it means she would be returning to the land her ancestors were stolen from, ushered by me. Except she believes it isn't yet time.

"This morning I spoke with my prayer group and they reminded me that God isn't finished with me yet. I'm not done with this life. I'm not ready to die. I am going to be healed of this cancer!" She punctures the air around her bed with her finger on each accented syllable.

I am surprised, but the jovial nature of her home suddenly makes more sense. I wasn't expecting this, and my bemusement has turned to curiosity. According to Reggie, I am here because she wants to create rituals for her deathbed. Akua knows what type of work I do and has asked for me specifically. From his description, she has been living with osteosarcoma for a few years already, but has been confined to her bed for months now and is aware her death is approaching. He tells me she's made peace with it. The tumor on her spine has grown rapidly, blocking the nerves that allow her to move her legs, and the cancer has metastasized to her brain. She is quite thin and frail; her dark brown eyes are shadowed by her brow bone. But they twinkle.

The week prior, Reggie and Akua had been looking for hospices and asked for my opinions based on the doctor's recommendation. Her time to die is approaching, but Akua is not ready. And it is not my job to convince her. I'm a death doula who believes in miracles, but still just a death doula. Not God. And God has told her that it isn't yet her time. I don't make it a practice to argue with what any god has told someone. That's a losing argument. Since death denial is often rooted in fear, I ask Akua what she's afraid of.

After some consideration, she replies softly, "That I will die before I have done all I need to do." This is a common fear of death. Death can come at any time, whether or not we are prepared, and we feel powerless at the notion. We think of our lives as our own, our egos wrapped up in what we have to contribute to the world, and not of ourselves as just one note in a symphony. When it's time, death doesn't fail.

"I am a dancer and a performer, you see, and I still have my best work before me." Her conviction is so pure I want to believe her. She still dances with her arms along with the music and her words, Fela's saxophones now a whisper in the background.

"What would you like to do in the time you have left?" I ask. It seems like a safe enough question. I hope she doesn't notice that I have neither affirmed nor denied her suggestion.

"I want to surround myself with music and art. I want to dance again. I want to write plays and perform on stages. There is still art in me." Together we conceive of what the next few months could look like, making alternate plans for the possibility that the tumor on her spine doesn't allow her to dance. I fear she will never dance again, but for a moment, I keep this to myself.

I struggle with this decision. Am I feeding a delusion that Akua will eventually be back on the stage? Hope, at the end of life, is double-edged: it can either be a powerful motivator or it can blind us to the truth we must prepare for. We might reasonably hope to make it to our granddaughter's graduation, but hoping for a miracle when science and the reality of our dying bodies tells us different? That can be crushing. I want to guard Akua from the disappointment that will eventually come when her cancer spreads. It is my understanding that it is spreading quickly. But I can't save her (or anyone) from the deep pain of embracing her mortality. If I tell Akua what I believe to be the truth, she might crumple under the weight of it. She might shut down. But it might also mean that she is better prepared to face what is coming.

This is a classic death doula's dilemma but with only one solution: meet the client where they are. In their journey toward death, I remind each human of their right to make their own choices. Akua chooses to dream of dance. At that moment, I choose to dream with her.

We agree that I will find her a wheelchair that can fit through her doorway and look for a contractor to put a small ramp at the entrance to her apartment building so she can get into a wheelchair vehicle. She wants to go to shows, so we look at the schedule for the Ahmanson Theatre in Los Angeles, her favorite venue. I don't feel any internal conflict supporting her in this. I am not promising Akua that she will recover fully. I am supporting her in living these days in the way that will fill her spirit. This is the highest creed of a death doula.

In the next two weeks, Akua and I speak every few days. The wheelchair is easy to acquire. The ramp down the front steps of her apartment building is not. The contractor is willing, but the building isn't ADA compliant. That's a battle that I am clear we don't have time for. Her disease is progressing and in a short time, the tumor on her spine will continue to spread pain throughout her body. Reggie, after his initial shock and frustration that his mom has been insisting she would recover, calls again and asks me to go back. This time, he assures me, Akua wants to talk about her death.

My heart hurts for him. He is a mother's son, terrified about losing her and also what it would mean for her to die without making peace with her ending. If Akua had been my own mother—and with her smooth brown head, bald from years of chemo, and her Christian convictions, she reminded me of her—I might have been more impatient with her dreams. But she is not. Tash taught me that.

The next time I visit Akua, there is no Fela Kuti playing, but the heaps of items and art still decorate the floor of her apartment. Her closet doors are open and her bed faces the rows of colorful clothing. "Take whatever you want," she says, gesturing weakly at the display. Never mind that the last time I was her size I was six years old, and even then I was probably rounder than she ever was, healthy. I oblige and go through Akua's closet, using the opportunity to talk about what she wore and what she's seen in her life. She tells me stories of the costumes, the productions she's been in, and the seamstress in Ghana who made an outfit for her out of traditional kente cloth. This time she sounds more like a woman who knows the end of her life is near—thoughtful, retrospective, and pensive, yet still dramatic. We don't lose all the parts of ourselves because we are dying. We become more of who we are.

When the style talk stops, Akua and I talk about her dreams of the Ahmanson Theatre. I apologize if I created any additional hope. Blaming no one but herself, she tells me that she willfully ignored the doctors, the referral for hospice, and the pain coursing through her body. She wasn't yet ready. But in her quiet moments, she'd begun to consider what her tumor has come to teach her.

When she accepted the truth that her death was around the corner, she'd connected with what she most wanted out of her life: dance, performance, the stage. When it was clear she wouldn't get to *do* it anymore, she looked for ways to *be* it. She shared that her tumor had come to remind her that she was a dynamic and resplendent being regardless of whether she was on a stage. It was her birthright and she no longer needed to be on the stage to claim it. She had lived it. And now she is ready to consider her deathbed and to die.

For Akua's death, she wants to be surrounded by purple roses, lilacs, and lilies. She wants to hear Nils Frahm playing on the speakers, as loud as her dying body can bear. She wants us to close her chakras as she is actively dying, and together we create a ritual to complete after she has released her last breath. She wants Reggie, his wife, her grandchildren, and her best friend present with her. She wants to be in her home, which is alive with music, art, and experiences. But most important, she wants to die in full surrender, grateful for the gift to have been resplendently and dynamically human. Her death came just three weeks after my first visit, and a few days after my last.

Had we tried to force Akua to embrace her death earlier, she likely wouldn't have made this powerful self-discovery. She did it in her own time. Sometimes all we need is a little time, if we've got it. And for others to lovingly hold us exactly where we are. And if you're the person who can't accept that another will die, we will hold you when you finally do.

Chapter 6

Teach Me How to Doula

Most people, at some point in their lives, will serve as a death doula. Living and dying in community means at some point a member of our community will need the support—a grandparent, neighbor, best friend, a pet. If it were up to me, everyone would have a functional death literacy—an understanding of the importance of it, tools to support another, insights on how to sit with our mortality, and skills. Lots and lots of skills.

Compassion and service are at the root of my work. But those forces alone don't make you a death doula. Being a death doula requires more than sitting bedside, holding hands, and singing "Kumbaya."

An effective death doula must pay deep attention to their own relationship to death, along with their inherited judgments, biases, privileges, and limitations. We must understand the bureaucracy and legalities surrounding dead bodies, have a vast base of information and resources, and be able to work alongside care teams. It is useful to be as well-versed in the practicalities of preparing for death as in the arts of ritual creation, holding multiple truths, and navigating emotional depth. And we must do it all while honoring our needs.

This is essentially what we learn in death doula training, even though there is no formal school. It is an art, a craft. This work is as ancient as humankind. For as long as people have been living, others have been supporting them through their deaths.

Not every death doula takes a training course. Some learn this work through their lineage, or sitting at the feet of the community member who is called when death is occurring. Most of us are just thrown into it, as I was with Peter.

In the months after Peter's death, I let grief guide me. It was a tough period. One of deep sorrow but also of burgeoning curiosity. I wondered how the sun kept coming up. I would burst into tears or laughter at socially inappropriate times. I wore Peter's T-shirts and leather jacket. I read every book about death that I could get my hands on. The veil was thin. No matter where I looked, I could easily see how life and death interacted.

I wasn't sure if it was just a grief response or a fleeting interest, as I'd had so many of them. But since my desire to be closer to the dying persisted, I sought out a training program, recommended to me by my therapist.

She mentioned a woman she knew who had taken an Introduction to Death Midwifery course at a place with the intriguing name Sacred Crossings. She gave me her email address on a sticky note.

"Who knows?" she said. "Give it a whirl."

She didn't know how serious I was yet. I put my vitriol for sticky notes aside and guarded it like it was a million dollars.

Sacred Crossings is both an alternative funeral home and a death education organization. Their upcoming intro session was already full, but I begged and pleaded with the instructor over the phone, promising to bring my own cushion, water, and snacks. She relented.

When I knocked on the door at the Pacific Palisades house where the session took place, I was greeted by a gorgeous woman with soft brown shoulder-length hair wearing a velvet kimono and a scarf named Olivia Bareham. "You're quite persistent," she said, laughing in a singsong British accent and regarding me quizzically.

"You've got no idea!" I replied, cheesing brightly. Instantly warm,

Olivia welcomed me into the living room. There were three beige, textured couches packed with people, while others had opted for colorful floor cushions, meditation stools, or lotus positions on the rugs on the hardwood floor.

For an hour I listened to the work of death midwives. "I wanted to wash and dress my husband's body after his death, but the nurses told me that the funeral home should do it," said an older white woman with close-cropped gray hair and turquoise and coral jewelry. Another soft-spoken older woman mentioned that after her husband's death, his body was gone within half an hour. She didn't know that bodies could be kept at home, and she would have opted to have a little more time with him had she'd known. Around the room, the other participants nodded.

Every person in the room seemed like a variation on these two— older, overwhelmingly white, silver-haired, lots of scarves and tie-dye. Nonetheless, there was no doubt that these were my people. All of us felt the pull toward that inky, dense, indescribable moment in human life, the terminus point that gives life its meaning. On my way out I grabbed a handful of brochures on the table and skipped to my car. I got in, snapped my seat belt, and sobbed, laughed, cried, and danced in my seat. I knew I'd found something worth holding on to.

The Sacred Crossings Death Midwifery Program took place over three weekends in 2014. Patrick and I were traveling a lot then to help nurse my grief after Peter's death. So during the course, I'd fly in from whatever country I'd set up a temporary home in, and get my mind and heart blown open by Olivia and my fellow students for a few days, before settling in with a stack of books.

The Tibetan Book of Living and Dying by Sogyal Rinpoche put words to the ephemeral nature of life and the ineffable awe I experienced as Peter died. *It's OK to Die* by Dr. Monica Williams-Murphy and Kristian Murphy highlighted the bankrupting of America through the injustice of its healthcare system, showing me that my advocacy had a place in this world too. *Ritual* by Malidoma Some reminded me that a sacred life is a ritualized life, which helps us prepare for death. I was starting to learn the truth about my chosen path: death work, like death itself, was unfathomably vast. I could tunnel forever and still be no closer to the mystery.

I finished the course one year after Peter died, despairing that we didn't have access to this information to make his dying gentler on all of us. I was clear now: if it were up to me, every person on earth would have the support that I now knew was possible.

Early on, I wanted to know how to build out a practice that extended beyond caring for bodies at home and home funerals. I wanted to understand the logistical side as well. I got a part-time job at an alternative funeral home called Friends Funeral Home and Cremations with a woman named Ziri Rideaux. I volunteered at Tranquil Care Hospice and worked to help build Anam Cara, a rare social model hospice home in L.A. County, which sought to house people who lacked the support to die in their own homes or who were in need of a place to die. I also got a license to sell life insurance so that I could understand how it worked. I interrogated and bought coffee and cake for so many people who worked in death-adjacent industries, including estate planning attorneys. I wanted to understand the work they did, as it was a different area of law from the ones I practiced at Legal Aid. I kept their business cards handy to give to clients who needed the support. That's as far as I engaged my legal background in crafting my doula business. Once I was done with the practice of law, I never looked back.

Going with Grace was formalized in 2015 after a ten-day Vipassana silent meditation retreat where the name and business structure dawned on me. Of the people most surprised that I built a capable business, I am at the top of the list. I never had a mind for it. I bristle at capitalism, give things away all the time, and got fired from any job where I had to sell anything. But I knew in this job, I wouldn't have to convince anyone of anything. I just needed to share what was on my heart, and there was a lot on it.

I shared my idea with a friend I'd met at a hospice volunteer training named Emily Marquez, who was as excited about it as I was. We dove in headfirst together. Emily would handle the marketing; I would handle the content. We brainstormed ideas, tried out fonts, and tried writing a business plan. After six months, we decided to part ways, but Going with Grace as it stands would never have existed without Emily. With her blessing, I pushed forward, terrified to be going it alone. I had to do it scared.

With my business structure set, the spark I felt in Cuba on the bus with Jessica turned into a little fire, gaining flames as I learned more about the experiences of others. Being in the trenches with Peter had made it personal. I was still angry but I was also hungry. I knew I was embarking on a line of work that touches every human being on the planet and every aspect of society. How would I ever get bored?

Building a business as a death doula, though, *was* boring. I didn't know the first thing about it, but I had no choice. My laptop became my best friend, but the clingy, energy-vampire kind. There's a digital photo album of me from those years titled "today's office looks like," and it's not glamorous: me and my laptop on a Long Island Rail Road train, in cabs, at coffee shops, at the mechanic's, at a bar during happy hour with friends nearby. Inspiration struck everywhere, so I'd work on content, create workshops, research tax rules, mock up promotional materials, and draft cold intro emails everywhere. There was no "off" switch for me.

After I formalized the business, I hung out a shingle and waited for clients.

None came.

So I set out to find them. I took meetings at hospices in Los Angeles, but most doors were shut in my face by folks who felt I was encroaching on their territory. The consensus at the time was that I either didn't understand hospice or was an excitable kid whose passion would soon run out. I felt like a door-to-door encyclopedia salesperson.

One hospice, thank the god of Abraham, offered me a place in their Death Day event in the parking lot next to their building. I set up a white folding table with turquoise saree fabric I'd bought in India, and spread my business cards and brochures on the desk. Standing awkwardly and fidgeting in my turquoise African-print skirt to match the fabric, I handed out brochures I had printed for $2 each and smiled eagerly at each passerby, who probably wondered why I was so happy to be at a death event. When someone tossed their brochure in the trash after leaving my table, I went to retrieve it, smoothed it out, and put it right back on the table. Money was tight.

A couple I met at the Death Day event referred me to their friend whose mother was dying. I tried to keep my face solemn but inside I was doing cartwheels. *Someone was dying that wanted my support! Whee!* We did the consultation and she paid me double what I asked. She placed a higher monetary value on the service than I did. It was my first inkling that my business might work.

I held workshops for friends and family at first, then word spread. Soon, I was hosting a workshop every two weeks for about seven to ten people I didn't know. This was another terrifying new challenge: learning to speak in front of people about their mortality. I'd watched my parents preach in pulpits my entire life and could mimic their pauses, inflections, and emotional beats as an inside joke with my sisters. But when I had to open my mouth to address a crowd as *myself,* sometimes I heard those damn speech therapists trying to convince me that there was something wrong with the way I spoke. So when a chaplain friend of mine, Rev. Maggie Yenoki, offered me her pulpit at her Unitarian Universalist church to speak to her congregation about death, I was terrified—of not knowing what to say, of seeming like a death-obsessed weirdo, of being on display, of being vulnerable. Fortunately, with the strong urging of palliative care physican B. J. Miller, whom I met at one of his talks, I considered that I could reach more people at one go on a stage than I could one-on-one. And damn if he wasn't right. I got over myself, did the talk, and didn't burst into flames when I stepped into the pulpit. After that, I talked about death and dying wherever anyone would listen. Word about me and my services continued to spread.

At parties, I'd talk about my doula work and people would look at me funny. Either they would respond by wishing I were there when their mother/great-uncle/father/sister-in-law/pet tarantula died, launch into their ideas about the afterlife, or mutter "that's nice" and stay away from me for the rest of the party, eyeing me suspiciously from across the room. I wanted to tell them that I wasn't contagious. But maybe my passion was.

My own friends and family were intrigued by the work, but understandably hesitant. This wasn't my first time passionately declaring a new venture. When Bozoma picked me up from the airport in Peter's maroon Mitsubishi Eclipse on my return trip from Cuba, I shared my encounter with Jessica and my desire to get closer to death. She scrunched her face at me: "What the fuck happened to you in Cuba?" I giggled. My dad was hesitant, encouraging me to reconsider law, but I couldn't bring myself to do it. My mother, as always, said, "Oh, okay," which signified that she wasn't totally on board, but wasn't going to try to stop me. On the contrary, she let me share her one-bedroom apartment when I was broke, until I was finally able to chip in enough for us to afford a two-bedroom.

I like to believe that my loved ones withheld judgment because they saw a fervor in me that had been missing for a long time. I saw it too, and it felt amazing. Yet beneath my excitement lay raw fear: there was no blueprint to follow in death work. I didn't know of any existing businesses like mine. I didn't yet understand that entrepreneurship would be a spiritual journey—an unrelenting test of my faith in myself and my vision. I *knew* it was possible, but I had no evidence. Every day the questions nagged: Could this business really be viable? Does anyone give a shit except for me? Who was I to think that I could take this on? And am I cut out for it?

If I'd known then just how much death doula work would require of me, I might have gotten scared, thrown it all away, and become a nail tech. Death work is a perilous metaphysical high-wire act, and it will take you to places inside yourself you might not be ready to visit.

There have been clients over the years whose deaths filled me with so much light and life that I was flying, and deaths that were so challenging that they threw me back on my heels. They asked everything of me, drew upon every resource at my disposal. In those moments, I have been filled with the terror of not knowing if I had served them as they needed to be served. And then, when it was over, I would be left with crippling doubts. This didn't only happen when I was a fresh death doula either.

Six years into my business, I meet Justina. She is a well-known self-help guru who could have asked for anything on her deathbed, even looking at the *Mona Lisa* surrounded by hot Frenchmen. I am honored to get the call to support her in her death, which is only twelve days away, though of course we don't know that yet.

In our exploratory phone call, she shares that she is very ill from ALS and colon cancer, knows she is close to death, and wants to ensure her practical affairs are handled. When I walk in for our first meeting, I am greeted by an assistant who knows how to pronounce my name—a first. Everything about Justina's home rings true of what I've heard. Her front parlor is covered in fur rugs and Swarovski crystals. Little white Pomeranian dogs run around with a dedicated dog walker chasing them. A lush white throne with gold upholstery tacks sits in the corner. Glamour shots of her through the years are framed in gilded gold and decorate the walls. Her assistant points me through a set of French doors.

Through them, Justina sits in an armchair covered in old sheets, facing the television with no fewer than fifteen people sitting around her. Her hair is curled and brushed, lipstick poppin', nails done. She welcomes me cheerfully. People buzz in and out, bringing flowers, stories, and gratitude. She has a smile and a personal acknowledgment for every one. I start to understand why she is so beloved. Justina makes people feel seen. They thrive in her gaze.

We talk about what Justina needs and set baseline expectations for our work together. Aside from the adoring fans, this is a typical first meeting. Justina wants to update her will (No thanks. I connect her with an estate-planning attorney colleague), and needs help planning multiple public memorial services, including one at the famous Beverly Hills Hotel. I ask her what is still undone in her life, aside from practical matters. With an arrogant tilt of her head, she says, "Nothing." We speak of her four marriages. She says she'd had enough sex for seven lifetimes and grills me about my love life, wishing the same for me. I smile and joyfully receive the blessing of an OG like herself, but I wonder if she is dodging my question with juicy distractions.

Justina has reconciled her romantic relationships, she insists, but there's a sadness in her bright blue eyes I can't quite put my finger on, beyond existential dread. It nags at me. We finish the meeting by talking through her desired deathbed rituals, the songs she wants to hear as she's dying, and her thoughts about the afterlife.

On my second visit with Justina one week later, things have changed dramatically. The lipstick and the visitors are gone, and there is a heaviness in the air. The sorrow in her watery blue eyes is stark. We'd planned to talk about the disposition of her body and care of her pets, but it is clear she is not up for it. She's frustrated about an itch on her calf that her caregivers can't scratch to her satisfaction. She murmurs curses at them and at the sky. "No one understands. No one understands," she repeats quietly through tears. And she's right. We can't. People surround her daily, singing her praises. Numerous people live in her home and provide around-the-clock care for her, yet still she feels alone. She is the one facing her mortality.

As a hospice nurse tinkers with Justina's feeding tube, Justina wiggles her fingers at me, eyes pleading. I grab her hand and she squeezes it lightly as her eyes well up. It becomes clear that I am here not only to help make logistical plans. Justina wants me to journey with her, in this last stage of her life. When her nurse is finished, Justina orders everyone out, but asks me to stay. We sit in silence until it becomes solace.

Justina has been laid emotionally bare—a rarity for her as far as I can tell. In this state, she is harsh and dismissive of her caregivers. Her head hangs low, and she avoids eye contact with everyone she speaks to except me. She's not making jokes about her lovers, nor is she turning the questions on me. This is another side of her I have the honor of meeting—vulnerable, cracked open by illness.

Justina confesses that she is miserable and asks me to tell her how quickly she can expect to die. No answers I give can assuage her anguish. She tells me she doesn't want to bear this much longer. It's been two years of disease.

Though she has trouble communicating, she talks a lot. She is tired of the dozens of people milling about her home, whom she feels she has to smile for. She doesn't want to take her medication any longer, but doesn't feel free to communicate that to her doctors or caregivers. She feels like she owes it to her fans to keep living, to keep fighting, but she is tired. She reveals to me in a whisper that she has already gotten medication to end her life but doesn't know if she will take it. She wants no more visitors, no more deliveries, no half-strangers crying at her side. She wants to die surrounded by only the six people who know her best, whom she can be completely herself around, on her own terms.

This is critical for me to hear. It helps me identify Justina's most intimate needs of being seen, heard, and treated as a whole being. Justina's initial agitation has lifted. I leave that meeting clear about what I am there to do. I am there to support Justina in having an intimate death, not one witnessed by the world. I am there to manage the process, to honor her vulnerability, and to hold her for who she is—not who she is to me or to the adoring fans.

As Justina moves into the active dying phase a few days later,

I call the list of six people she has requested. However, word gets out that she is dying, so dozens of people show up, lurking around in the living room waiting to get their moment. It is like she is in a death zoo, with voyeurs trying to get the last little pieces of her while she is still living. It is a juggling act to hold space for their grief while also respecting Justina's wishes. I do the best I can, and still feel like I am failing.

This was not supposed to be happening. People fling themselves crying on her body or hold on to her feet while sobbing. I want to tell them to back off her, but I leave them there for a beat, then help them up and walk them behind a folding screen we'd put up to try to protect Justina's dying space. As soon as I move one person away, another sneaks in behind me.

Things get worse. Someone has taken down the folding screen, leaving her in full view. I enlist the hospice nurse like a bouncer to keep people away from Justina as she starts to make her exit. Hospice nurses can be death doulas' best allies in this work and vice versa. We are an extension of care for each other: an extra set of hands, eyes, and ears. Noticing that Justina's breath is slowing, the hospice nurse nods at me. I can no longer pay attention to keeping out extra folks. I turn my focus solely on Justina. I take my place by the side of her reclined armchair and hold her hand.

We hold vigil as her breathing slows, singing songs she's requested and stroking her head. The hospice nurse comes closer, holding the perimeter around Justina and her chosen six friends, and together we count seconds between her breaths. When she is taking just four breaths a minute, we glance at each other. She is close. After she releases her last breath, we take a sacred pause. The room is still as the gravity of what has occurred dawns, silent except for a few muffled sniffs. I model reverence by not moving. Right after a death, there is nothing to do but to sit in honor of what has just occurred.

When rustling begins and the cries get louder, I place Justina's hand in the hand of one of her friends nearby and take the center of the room. Through halting speech, I acknowledge the magnitude of what we've just witnessed, encourage everyone to be gentle with themselves in their grief, and ask for privacy as we handle Justina's body before the funeral home arrives. I know the funeral home won't come until we call them, but I just want the folks to give us, and Justina, some space. They file out, shell-shocked—the show is over.

Finally, it is just us.

We take a collective exhale after I've closed the door. I hold a bowl of warm water with a few drops of lavender oil in it, so her best friends can wash her body as Justina requested. We sit with her body. Her friends tell absurd stories about her life and her lovers. They joke about her hard head and big vision. They stroke her hair and kiss her hands. And they hold their friend in a way that only those who know us best can hold us.

On the road home, I call my mother and cry so hard I can't see the road. For over eight hours, I haven't taken a moment to myself, haven't had a sip of water, or a bite to eat. All of my focus has been on trying to keep Justina's death as intimate as she requested. My mother suggests I pull over until I gather myself, but I just want to be in my home, my sanctuary, so I call a car service to take me the rest of the way. I leave my car parked on a side street in L.A.

The rest of the day, I sit on the burnt-orange chaise lounge by the window in my apartment staring into the void, mindlessly eating kettle potato chips and crying. Something about the fat, salt, and crunch soothes me, particularly after I've attended a death. I am exhausted and regretful. I fear that I have failed Justina in her request only to have the people she most loved and trusted present at her bedside. That's not what she got.

Even after six years of practice, I wonder if I am cut out for this work.

After a few hours spent trying to make sense of what I experienced, I remember that I need to wash my body: a regular ritual when I get home from seeing a client. It engages my senses to ground me in my body and washes off what is not mine to keep. The thought of standing in the shower overwhelms me. Naked, I step into the bathtub but cannot figure out how to block the drain to take a bath even though I've done it dozens of times before. I cry out of frustration that I don't know how to care for myself at this moment. I call David, my boo of a year, and just tell him that I need him. I don't even know exactly what I need.

David comes over. He fills up the bathtub, adds Epsom salt and eucalyptus oil, and makes me a cup of tea while I soak. He sits on the toilet, listening as I pour out all my failures as a doula and my fears over my inadequacy to do this big work. He towels me off, and holds me while I talk and cry, and talk and cry, until I fall asleep. I am laid bare, snotty, and feeling like a failure.

A few days later, I begin to feel clarity again. In our session, the death doula students I am now teaching reflect back to me what I have shared with them about how to doula. They remind me that I held the differing experiences of both the grievers and the dying. I stayed grounded in the chaos. I worked with the medical care team. I honored my client's needs above all, and I honored my need to also be taken care of. And they remind me of the bulldozing and purifying power of witnessing a death.

"Failure," as I had conceived of it, was just another familiar demon rearing its head in my subconscious. Justina taught me to divorce myself from the experience. It was not about what I could do and what I could not. It was about *her* death. Justina had died in the arms of her closest friends, as she had asked. I had held her hand. I had served her. For people on their deathbeds, serving their needs is all we can do.

Chapter 7

Stay Black and Die

I start working with a client named Nancy in June 2016. She's a ninety-six-year-old white woman—a former librarian with an affinity for cats and succulents—who developed Alzheimer's fifteen years prior. Nancy's daughter has hired me to sit with her in the elder care facility where Nancy's spending the end of her life. Even though the staff is generally warm and understanding, these places often feel like warehouses for people to waste away as they descend into death. Often, they are the best a family can do.

Nancy's daughter realizes the additional social time my visits give her mother is valuable, even if—for whatever reason—she can't provide them herself. It is clear, though, that Nancy's daughter loves her mother, and is trying to provide her comfort.

And so I get to know Nancy over several months. This is not unusual in my death work. Some clients I work with for months, some for weeks, some for days, some just a hurried phone call.

At ninety-six, Nancy wants to be independent, but her brain and body no longer make that possible. She likes to take walks solo, but can't find her way back. The facility she's at has a locked unit to keep her from wandering beyond the doors where she will get lost. She can barely remember her daughter, let alone her way home. Each visit, I introduce myself anew and ask her if it is okay if I stay for a while because she has no recollection of our previous visits. With a coy, flirtatious smile, she always says, "Why yes," touching the barrette on the right side of her head and tucking her short but still-thick gray hair behind her ear.

Nancy's disease has progressed in the time we've been working together. At first, we could have a full conversation: we initially bonded over our mutual love of books. Nancy *loved* books (Agatha Christie's *And Then There Were None* was a favorite), not just reading them but their shape, smell, and physical presence. She could wax rhapsodic about the spine of a particular book in a way that made me love it too. We would stay with a topic for as long as she could before a non sequitur introduced a hard left, and I'd try to keep up.

After six weeks or so, conversation becomes harder; she forgets words, gets frustrated, and shuts down. Sometimes, we look through her books on birds and she tells me about them, or she shows off her photo albums. But at this point, she's forgotten who most of the people and birds are, again to her frustration. So we sing songs together, or I sit by her as she eats, entering into whatever reality she's currently inhabiting. Our visits are pleasant, and an exercise in going along for the ride.

About six months into our visits, I arrive to find her visibly agitated, a departure from her normal genteel demeanor. She sits alone at a table in the community room, stuffing balled up newspapers into the pockets on the side of her wheelchair while the corner television blares. Groups of elders sit at tables playing card games, reading, snacking, or staring off into space. Nancy occasionally pulls a sheet of newspaper off a stack on the table and tries to read it, but since her brain has atrophied long past the point of comprehension, she stares at it before angrily ripping it into pieces, which she then shoves back into her wheelchair pockets. She does this over and over again as fast as her arthritic hands will allow, but no one takes notice. Life in a long-term care home goes on around her.

Over Nancy's shoulder in the stack of newspapers, I spot an obituary for actress and socialite Zsa Zsa Gabor, who gained popularity in the early 1950s and had died just a few days before. Given that Alzheimer's patients in moderate stages of the disease can sometimes access long-term memory, I point at the picture to try to refocus Nancy's frenetic energy.

"Yes, yes, I know her!" Nancy says immediately.

I am surprised. "You do?"

"Yes, I do. She's in the pictures. She's so beautiful. So sweet." Nancy looks at the page and smiles affectionately. Her shoulders soften. I feel that maybe we've found a connection again through the static, despite her mood. After a minute, she squints at the page then picks it up, putting it right up to her face, as though she's discovered a secret code on it.

She turns her face up in disgust. "Is she *Black*?" The question is hurled like an accusation.

"Uhhhhh . . ." I stutter. As far as I know, Zsa Zsa Gabor is Eastern European—in other words, pretty damn white. I can see it plainly in her obituary photo and am surprised that Nancy is confused. I am so stunned that I can't get out an answer before she slams the paper down then turns her laser eyes on me.

"Wait, are *you* Black?" Again, the word *Black* is a dart shot at me.

I am dumbfounded. Speechless.

Of course I am Black.

I am Black *as fuck*.

When I identify myself, one of the first words I use is *Black*. I don't use the term African American because in its strict definition, it does not apply to me. My lineage is Ghanaian, and so the legacy of American slavery is not mine to claim. My ancestors were the ones whose villages were pillaged and burned, whose loved ones were beaten and stolen, and who were left to weep over their fates in West Africa. Technically, I am of a third culture—born African, raised in America, my family mixing the two to create our own.

Yet, when a white woman grabs her purse when I walk too fast around a corner, she does not know, nor does she care, that I am Ghanaian. Neither do I. It does not matter. She and I are both privy to her perception of me as a threat. Each of us with highly melanated skin living in the United States of America lives under that same cloud of racism, whether Ghanaian, Jamaican, African American, or Afro Brazilian.

Am I Black? she wants to know. Hell yeah I'm Black.

My mind races at the implications of Nancy's question. I want to ask a doctor if Alzheimer's can make people appear more hateful or simply unveils their true feelings, like alcohol unveiling desire and decreasing inhibition—Alzheimer's beer goggles. I doubt it. Thus far, Nancy's been pretty sweet with me, but I am aware that mood and personality changes are a symptom of the disease. Is Alzheimer's causing a kind of race blindness in this woman, revealing race as the false construct it is, or is it allowing her racist flag to fly freely?

Before I can figure out how to answer Nancy's question, she picks up the paper again and furiously starts tearing it to bits. My mind swirls with conjecture and fear. Nancy was born in 1920, which means her formative years happened during the Jim Crow era. For all I know, she may still believe Black people pollute swimming pools and come from monkeys. When she was growing up, lynchings were still common, as were sanctioned race-based violence and overt segregation. When Nancy was a girl, Black people were not even a full generation past slavery.

Up until that moment, I'd made a conscious choice to feel safe around her. She was ailing, and she needed my support, so I gave her the benefit of the doubt. It should not come as a surprise to me that as her mind regresses, she might say some wild shit. But it is the first time something like that has happened in my death work.

Among many things, what strikes me about this encounter with Nancy is that the inequities she lived through and benefited from would follow her into her death. I think not enough people realize this. I am exasperated that people believe death is the great equalizer. Yes, we all die, but we die of different causes at different rates in different ways. There is nothing equal about death, except that we all do it. Death and dying are culturally constructed processes that reflect social power dynamics—they are unequal. How we die is wrapped up largely in the intersections of our identities.

To adequately support people who are dying, we must be willing to look at their complex set of identities. White women live longer than Black women. Men die earlier than women. Straight people live longer than queer folks. Poor people die earlier than wealthy ones.

These are facts. We are not all born the same, and we do not live or die the same.

On average, Black American babies are born into a different set of circumstances than white American babies. The gap between the two continues through life and into death. Black bodies bear the deep scars of medicalized racism, systemic brutality, and intergenerational trauma.

There's also the added basic stress of living Black in America, which is created by trying to assimilate into a world which fears Black bodies. In tense moments, I know I stand a better chance of surviving conflict if I make myself small and unthreatening, and if I quiet myself down so that I am not deemed rowdy or scary.

This happens in personal, public, and professional settings. Before I worked for myself, I stayed quiet when work wasn't distributed fairly because I didn't want to seem angry. I don't go for walks at night when I have pent-up energy because I don't want to provoke neighborhood attention. To this day, I'm scared to get pulled over by the cops. The sheer number of ongoing stressors, big and small, that come with existing in this skin are too numerous to recount.

Yet here I am, a Black death doula, hoping to ease the difficulties we *all* face in death. My presence in this field is important, because when deathcare is done without awareness of difference, privilege, and bias, it can be used as a weapon, further marginalizing communities and people at one of the rawest, most excruciatingly painful moments of their lives.

This matters. It *matters*. In the same way people want their identities validated in life, they want that in death too. And it's crucial that their loved ones see it happen, as a sign of their beloved being seen, respected, and honored.

There is a sort of fake colorblindness that runs rampant in wellness spaces ("I don't see color" or "I forgot that you are Black") that sadly has found its way into the death and dying community as well. I can't trust or believe anyone who says they don't see color—unless they are actually blind. Their refusal to see *me* in all my glory serves as a refusal to acknowledge and appreciate my individualism and rich history. It's an oppressive erasure which does not acknowledge, among other things, that Black people's strength is evidenced by the ability to surrender without being broken. If I don't catch myself, it's easy to feel invisible in a field dominated by white people and stuck in systems that don't consider the privileges, prejudices, and biases that exist in every other place. If I had a dollar for every time someone said "I don't know what *race* has to do with how we die," I'd pay cash for a pimped-out G Wagon with rims.

As I said above: I am Black. As *fuck*. It is at the core of my identity. When everything else is stripped away, I'll still be proudly and loudly Black. I want that acknowledged when it's my time to go.

As a kid, I didn't have much of a concept of race. I could see the visual differences in humans, since we'd done a fair amount of traveling in my young life and I was exposed to a wide range of skin tones. When I was six, we moved from Orange, California—where my father was finishing up seminary—to Nairobi. My father had taken a position as the African director for Prison Fellowship International, opening up prison ministries in different countries in Africa. The apartment building we first moved into in Nairobi had Indian families, Irish families, other East Africans. I learned to judge people based on how giving they were. The Indian families were generous with cookies. Other families—the British, Ethiopian, and Ugandan—had children my age who would play with me and my sisters. One American family had rubber balls in every size, which we could take outside while the adults talked about adult things. Race was a foreign concept. The only yardsticks were generosity of spirit and snacks.

My parents enrolled my three sisters and me into one of the best schools in Nairobi, which included lots of the children of various missionaries in Kenya. They were also overwhelmingly white. (Apparently, the ability to leave your home country to travel and spread Jesus is a privilege.)

The classes at Rosslyn Academy were small and mostly segregated by age, except in music class, where younger and older students mixed. The music teacher assigned instruments every week, and competition for drums was fierce. I imagine that most of the students picked drums because they couldn't be that noisy in their homes. That included me. I *only* raised my hand for the drums. From one of the back rows, I'd jump up and down with my little hand in the air, hoping to be seen. One day, the teacher finally selected me. My heart did a little backflip at my good fortune.

I walked proudly (read: *boastfully*) toward the front of the room to claim my rightful place at the drums. As I did, I heard some whisperings. "Why her?" "She's Black." "Can she even *play* the drums?" Slowly, shame flooded in to replace my excitement. It started to dawn on me: my very existence made me different. *I am not like them. And what I am is something they don't like. And they think there is something wrong with me.* I wanted to cry in confusion, but beat my pain out on the drums instead.

Because of my parents' mission work, we never stayed in one place for long. Wherever we touched down, I learned that my Blackness meant something different. We returned to Ghana for a short stint a few years later, where race as a construct does not exist. In Ghana, everyone is Black, so no one has to be Black. There is nothing else to compare it to. I'm glad I had that experience before my family made the permanent move to America years later. It gave me a strong sense of myself before the complicated tentacles of racism began to prick my skin in ultraconservative, evangelical, terribly white Colorado Springs. I felt growing pride in my skin, lips, cheekbones, resiliency, and audaciousness.

And yet.

In my first week in school in sixth grade at Howbert Elementary, I was called a jungle bunny, an African booty scratcher, a monkey, and a fudgesicle. My sense of being the "other" was sharpened, and I grew arrogant to mask my hurt. It's hard enough to be the new kid halfway through a semester. It was almost unbearable to be one of the only Black kids, chubby, coming from a continent most of my peers looked down upon, while also being in the throes of puberty. My classmates asked if I rode elephants to school and if this was the first time I'd worn clothes. My mom still made our clothes. I liked it that way. I thought I was stylish, but hadn't yet learned how uncool it was not to have the newest Reeboks or Hammer pants. How dare they call me names when I'd seen more of the world by eleven years old than they would probably see in their lifetimes? They had never even been on a plane to leave the state, let alone travel the world. They didn't know of the skyscrapers, the toll roads, the electricity, the joy, the history, and the regality of Africa. I said nothing, but I knew they were the ignorant ones. It was humiliating.

My parents comforted me by modeling resilience. When it came to hurt and disappointment, my family's unspoken mantra was *Don't let them get to you.* Tears were allowed, but not indulged. The one time I remember crying uncontrollably was when a kid called me a "fat ugly brown cow" during a game of red rover. My mom told me he didn't understand my beauty, patted my back, and told me not to cry. I couldn't stop the tears. She let me cry it out.

We were the only Black family on our block, in our neighborhood, in the city, it seemed, so our home was an oasis. We spoke Fante there and almost exclusively ate Ghanaian food. No matter where we went, on Saturday afternoons my mom would line all four of her daughters up and do our hair: blue Ultra sheen pomade, hair baubles in every conceivable color tangled in with rubber bands. Combs of every size littering the floor. We'd sit between her legs, one by one, and she'd tug and pull, detangle, oil, condition, part, then braid us to Black girl perfection to get us ready for church on Sunday.

Meanwhile, school administrators tried to hold me back a grade given my lisp and the continent where most of my education happened. When my parents insisted that I be tested to see how I fared, the evaluators suggested that I skip two grades. I was considered "gifted," a label that followed and haunted me. How's that for an African booty scratcher?

Prioritizing my social development, my parents declined to skip me. Praise Yahweh. I felt like enough of an outsider as it was. I wasn't into what a lot of the other kids were into. Not feeling like the others hurt. I hurt a lot in those years.

Today, I see that being an outsider prepared me for my life in death work in ways that the girl in the "Out of Africa" spotlight in the yearbook could never have predicted. The dying, after all, are outsiders. They are on their way out of this life while the rest of us are steeped in it. We regard them as if through a pane of glass. I'm drawn to get close to it, to the place where people turn away because it is too frightening, too different, too scary. I don't think it's an accident that in my Going with Grace doula training classes, white cisgendered and heterosexual folks are sometimes in the minority. I can only remember three straight white guys in thousands of students who are otherwise queer as folk, inhabit many intersections, and celebrate their difference. Those who sit on the fringe in life can more easily get close to the fringe in death.

Still, there were bright spots in my adolescence. For every teacher who could only see my skin color and suggested I strongly consider becoming a secretary (even though I was in Advanced Placement English classes), there was someone like my choir teacher, Mr. Craig Ramberger, who encouraged me to apply to conservatories because he thought I had a lot of talent. I made friends, joined the cheerleading team, made homecoming court and MVP of the soccer team, and enjoyed music classes—early drumming experiences be damned.

Music provided a safe outlet for the big, messy emotions I'd already intuited were a little "too much" for the outside world. In choir, I could sing my feelings and let them go: Pachelbel's Canon in D made me feel so deeply I hid in the bathroom to cry, embarrassed by the depth of my emotional experience.

As much as I loved it, music as a career path was a no go. My parents instilled the belief in my sisters and me that we could be anything . . . as long as it was a doctor, a lawyer, or an engineer. Something prestigious and high-achieving, in other words, but nothing creative. Creativity didn't make money—always my father's biggest concern even though he played the clarinet and bought us recorders to practice on. He wanted to know that we'd be able to take care of ourselves as adults and take care of him when he got old.

After being accepted to a number of prestigious colleges—no thanks to my guidance counselor—I chose Wesleyan University, where my dad got his Ph.D. and where Bozoma was already enrolled. A small part of me still wonders who I would have become had I chosen Oberlin Conservatory. I might be a maestro living in Madrid sipping espressos all day, smoking skinny cigarettes and wearing faded skinny black jeans. I wonder if I also would have eventually found my way to death work. Different paths, same destination?

I chose Malcolm X House, the Black dorm, for my on-campus freshman-year housing. I wanted that feeling again from Ghana, where everyone was Black. The classes and students were a crash course in every piece of Black American culture I had missed in lily-white Colorado Springs—like bell hooks, dance hall reggae, and Spades. (I suck at Spades but stand on the side talking shit.)

Gradually, I understood that Blackness could look and sound like anything. It could mean my hilarious freshman-year roommate and forever best friend, Magda Labonté, a Haitian American Brooklynite actress and Libra who loved Mr. Cheeks from the Lost Boyz and wouldn't take an ounce of perceived disrespect from anyone. It could look like the Bay Area premed students who threw around the word *hella* and stressed about organic chemistry. It could look like Nigerian art students and Brazilian athletes. I could be a Black weirdo hippie and everybody was cool with it. Björk, plantains, and Biggie Smalls—all were my lanes.

So was activism. In 1998 I pledged a historically Black sorority dedicated to sisterhood, scholarship, and service—Delta Sigma Theta Incorporated Pi Alpha Chapter—and studied abroad in Ghana, where I was freshly enraged by the ravages of colonialism. Upon my return, I was elected student body president, running on a platform to support financial aid for students of color, to reduce the loan burden we carry after graduation. We graduate tens of thousands of dollars in debt, and then we spend decades trying to outrun the interest rates, barely touching the principal. We cannot buy homes or amass wealth even with our education, which is meant to even the playing field. We start in the red. The system is not set up for us to win. It shows up in different aspects of how we live, and it also shows up in how we die.

My anger continued, and my formal education gave me the tools to make people finally pay attention. I started to understand my power and supplemented it with my outward appearance. Black combat boots, camouflage pants, an African-print shirt I'd likely sewn, and a cowrie shell necklace were all in heavy rotation. Then I cut my hair off.

The "big chop," which rids a Black woman of all chemically processed hair, didn't become popular and mainstream until twenty

years later. But years of trying to fit into a white beauty standard had
exhausted me. Instantly, the barber was unhappy with my request.
"That haircut will make you look ugly," she observed. Internalized
racism is a bitch.

She asked if I'd had my heart broken. I said yes but not the way she
was suggesting. My heart had been broken by Amy in seventh grade,
who told me my worst features were my lips, my butt, how dark
my skin was even though she frequented tanning beds. My heart
was broken by *Seventeen* magazine's models, by teachers who refused
to see my intelligence because of my skin. My heart was broken by
America. I told the barber, again, to cut it off. My hair was going to
grow out of my head just as it came in. Coiled. Thick. Beautiful. And
brazenly Black as fuck.

There is almost no education about caring for Black people in
the deathcare industry, but on the slim chance some exists, it usually comes in the form of "Black hair care." This segment focuses on
caring for a tightly coiled hair pattern—as if this is the only "Black"
hairstyle, and not one of about *fifteen* different hairstyles that I alone
have had throughout my life.

How we define a good death is largely impacted by our identities. In conversation with a trans death doula student at Going with
Grace, they mentioned that they don't know what a good death could
be for them because they are scared to envision it for themselves. The
rate of violent death for trans folks is staggering, and this student
just doesn't want to be murdered. Yet when imagining what a "good
death" could be for a cisgender, heterosexual, white person, it can
come effortlessly.

We are conditioned to think of a "good death" as one that happens
at an old age, in our own home, surrounded by our loved ones, after
full peaceful lives, having our humanity acknowledged and honored
at the end of life. Most of the good deaths we think of are those in
which the body slowly shuts down.

Historically, however, Black people have died a great number of "bad" ways—at the hands of those that kidnapped and captured them, in the dungeons packed upon each other, in the transatlantic slave trade, at the hands of slave owners; through beatings, government experimentation, street violence, police brutality; in childbirth, in the carceral complex; and from a host of other conditions in the body, as a result of systemic racism. These epigenetic traumas take root in the family tree, passing down from generation to generation. But generational joy is also our birthright.

Many of the attributes that we think of in the "good death" are the same attributes that create a good life. But everybody is different. Every body. The myth of a Black monolith, in death, as in life, robs us of our quirks, our humor, our loves, our obsessions, our individuality, and our intersections. I think it's an attempt to make Blackness easier to understand and digest. But you cannot reduce us. How do you generalize about a race of people that has endured centuries of brutalization and still refused to have their joy suppressed?

Acknowledging this truth is the best way to achieve that elusive good death, which is based on who we were as individuals, and not as a monolith.

We all deserve that.

Chapter 8

Finding Your Feet

Falling in love sometimes feels like tripping over yourself. It's one of life's big messy adventures, and one of my greatest joys. Over a lifetime of relationships, I've become a connoisseur of its many stages. That deep belly-tickle at discovering rapport with a promising stranger—the hint of recognition, the surge of chemicals. Ooooh, he *cute*-cute. Then their intoxicating smell, slowly becoming familiar; the whisper of a private nickname as lips brush the ear. The gradual softening into a relationship, as falling in love expands into *love,* the enduring kind. The body, heart, and psyche are forever changed, and that love stays on in us till we die.

Falling in love can create a paralyzing fear of death. We become so much more aware of our mortality and that of our beloved when we are in love. We fear losing them, and life holds more value and purpose. It can be terrifying. But what else matters except opening ourselves to love? It's one of the "whys" of life. It shapes our fullest, most vivid memories. And its ultimate loss feels like an unmendable rupture. When a loved one dies, their love for you and your love for them doesn't go anywhere. It just changes form.

I've declared undying love for a solid number of the people I've dated, and even some strangers (like Tevin Campbell). My friends and family mostly roll their eyes at me: *Here she goes again.* I laugh off their teasing and try to ignore their implicit judgments. Like that I run hot and cold, that I am a flirt, that I am flighty, that the love I feel—and express—is somehow less profound or less meaningful than the adult, "real" kind of love.

Love doesn't look like one thing. Some of us feel it, in its purest form, in a series of encounters; others in long-term relationships. For some, monogamy is a sacred covenant. For others, it can be a jail. However you come by genuine love, you should take it and you should give it. My people might tease me for how fiercely I seize love when it is available. But my love declarations have been real. Every time. No matter how it ends. Because eventually my lover will die, as will I.

When Kip walked into my life, I had just arrived out west with my juris Doctor from University of Colorado Boulder School of Law shoved into my bags. I was in Los Angeles visiting my cousin Tina for a few days before I began my post–law school "adult" life in Oakland. I stopped at a gas station in Hollywood to fill up my green Honda Accord after the drive from Colorado, and he was across the pump filling up his green Ford Explorer. Our vehicles were similar hues and, seeking a way to move from sly glances and smiles to conversation, he commented on it.

He was six-two, dark-skinned, and buff, with skinny locs that fell all the way down his back and eyebrow and tongue rings that gave him an intriguing edge for an eighth-grade English teacher. (If he'd been *my* eighth-grade English teacher, I would have failed over and over again just so I could stare at him.) We realized he was born exactly one week before me. We felt like kindred spirits.

He was so many things in one: a sneaker head with an immaculate collection of Jordans in every color and style. A musician, producing funky beats for hungry young rappers out of his makeshift, in-home music studio, which was as pristine as his closet's perfectly arranged sneaker collection. On our first date, he took me to Toi Thai on Sunset Boulevard. I had pad thai with a side of brown rice, which I ate with a spoon in one hand and fork in the other, like I'd learned while living in Thailand for a summer. He marveled at my agility. I ate too much because I was nervous. He ate almost nothing, because he was nervous too.

We got into a conversation with our waiter about then-president George W. Bush. Our waiter was a fan; Kip was not. I pretended to be offended by Kip's sweeping generalizations about the Republican Party; he missed my sarcasm. When it dawned, he threw his head back and let out a thunderous baritone laugh, scrunching up his nose and shaking his head. By the time the mango sticky rice dessert came, I had hearts in my eyes.

Not wanting the date to end, we drove to the beach in Santa Monica, where we walked and held hands in the moonlight. We ranked our favorite albums and shared our beliefs about the world. That first night, we made a pact that regardless of whether or not the relationship worked out, we would still combine our DNA and have children, knowing that our genes would create superathletes. He believed we'd get rich with a son in the NFL. I didn't want kids, but making this playful pact with Kip was easy. He was stupid-cute, and his imagining a future with me was flattering. He was the kind of guy you usually only see in romantic comedies.

After only a few, sweet kisses, I got back to my cousin Tina's apartment at 3 A.M. and woke her up, feverishly announcing that I was going to marry Kip. My cousin groaned and rolled over, saying that she'd heard it from me before. (Which was true.) But one month after I arrived, I moved into Kip's apartment. Just like that, the life I had envisioned in the Bay Area disappeared.

I'd arrived in Cali on the strength of a coin flip. After graduating, all I knew was that I didn't want to go the fancy law firm route, even if one year's salary at one of those places could have decimated my student loan debt. I knew I wouldn't have been able to stomach all the golf, the money talk, and bullshit. I didn't care about the cases those places litigated, and I wouldn't be able to sleep at night knowing the role I played in them, however small. Now that I knew the broke lawyer's life was calling me, the only thing left to decide was whether to be a broke lawyer in New York City (so many friends, but *winter*) or somewhere in the state of California (no friends, but *sunshine*). Unable to choose, I resorted to chance: Heads, New York. Tails, California.

Cali won.

I settled on Oakland—centralized city life, plenty of liberals, hippies, queer folks, artists, and activists. After bland-ass Colorado, Black-ass Oakland would feel like the promised land.

Instead, I was nearly four hundred miles away in a 650-square-foot apartment in Pasadena with Kip. It might not have been what I'd planned, but what did that matter? We were blissfully happy.

Whenever we had small disagreements, he would apologize by writing me cute little songs. We had date nights in our apartment or on the roof, where he'd carry a table, chairs, candles, and speakers, and cover the ground with rose petals. When I had a disproportionate meltdown believing that a neighbor had stolen my computer and would sell it for parts, he laughingly reminded me that I was on hormonal birth control for the first time and perhaps the pills weren't working with my body chemistry. He was right, and I was angry that he was right.

The next few years were filled with the growing pains of young love as we stumbled our way through the "real" world. Kip made eighth-grade English teacher money in an underfunded public school, and although I wanted to help pay the bills, I put off finding a legal job for as long as I could. Instead, I worked as an extra on film sets, a front-desk person at a spa, and as a receptionist at a gym, where men trying to flirt asked me if I was an actress or model.

"Nope!" I would reply brightly. "I'm a lawyer."

Finally, I got a job at the Legal Aid Foundation of Los Angeles.

There it is, I thought with a stab of pride and a little dread. *I'm finally a proper lawyer.*

As the woman moving into Kip's bachelor pad, I introduced him to the revolutionary concept of shower caddies and dish towels. There was no couch, just an IKEA-grade futon facing a disproportionately large flat-screen TV that swallowed the opposite wall. When he built a sound booth in our bedroom, leaving me with no space for my shoes, I moved out into my own apartment. Eventually, he bought us a town house, which we renovated along with his father, nailing floorboards down and screwing in light fixtures. We stumbled our way forward, getting a lot of love right, and getting a whole lot of relationship wrong. We kept going.

After three years, the inevitable and annoying questions from family and friends began. When would we get married? When would we start a family? We were the "right" age—both twenty-nine—and from the outside we were the perfect couple: young, gifted, and Black, a lawyer and a teacher, both in public service. However, we were two very different people who were starting to discover that we didn't have the tools to negotiate a mutually agreed upon life.

Kip was a devout Christian and a homebody who preferred to spend Friday nights working on his music, grabbing dinner, and watching a movie. My ideal Friday nights were spent at concerts and socializing with fellow weirdos, twirling in the street, and letting *yes* lead the way. Although I too had a Christian upbringing, the Bible I kept—engraved and gifted to me by my parents on my eighteenth birthday—sat on my shelf alongside Maya Angelou, Hafiz, Osho, Carlos Castañeda, Eckhart Tolle, a biography of Jimi Hendrix, and *Tantric Orgasm for Women*. He dreamed of grandchildren running around us as we sat on a porch sipping lemonade. I dreamed of sipping Sauvignon Blanc in the Seychelles with him and my books. Despite our first-date pact to create superathlete offspring, the idea of raising children unnerved me and I communicated that, taking back my pledge early and often. It was clear we would not be able to form a cohesive life without some serious compromise. But we kept going.

When he asked me to marry him on the side of the 105, I grabbed the ring and instinctively sprinted down the freeway—laughing, crying, scared. We went home, cuddled in bed for a while, then called our families. I couldn't stop staring at my pretty new yellow sapphire and conflict-free diamond ring through the tears of joy. I was going to marry my best friend. I should have listened to my body, which ran when he asked the question. The body always wins.

Sorting through my feelings confused me. I *did* want to wear a pair of hot-pink Badgley Mischka crystal-encrusted heels and a fancy dress someday. But I felt feverish and wanted to peel off my skin at the thought of a wedding. I struggled to understand why we needed to throw a massive party for friends and families to honor a commitment we'd only make to each other. The compromise was that we'd elope to Costa Rica and the Casa del Sol Resort. I went barefoot on the beach in a borrowed dress and a bouquet of yellow and orange Gerbera daisies that my mother insisted upon. No Badgley Mischkas for me this time.

One Sunday afternoon when making our bed three months after we came back from Costa Rica, I learned that Kip didn't make the bed with a flat sheet. He preferred just the fitted sheet covering the mattress and a comforter. This was news to me, and I looked at him like he'd grown a snout. Would I have to live without a flat sheet for the rest of my life? Was I destined to a life of bacteria and skin cells absorbed directly into the comforter? What kind of life would that be? From there, my thoughts spiraled all the way out to my dreams of living in rural Japan, dancing in the falling cherry blossoms and drinking jasmine tea. Would I have to give all of that up? What other things would I have to compromise for the sake of merging my life with his? What other parts of me would have to die?

This innocuous tidbit threw me into a tailspin, unaware as I was that I was actually grieving my single life. Marriage was a mind fuck. I'd stare intently at him while he slept, trying to picture him as an old man. I couldn't. I cried silent tears into the pillow. I wanted to make him happy and I wanted to be happy, but I didn't know how to do both without losing myself in the process. I didn't have the language for it, but the long shadow of loss was creeping over me.

Despite couples therapy, we struggled. Kip was patient, but in the end, we couldn't figure it out. Six months after we stood across from one another on the beach, we agreed to separate. We had never filed the paperwork to register our marriage legally. When we fell apart, all that was required was for each of us to walk away.

The separation was excruciating, grim, and messy. At times it felt like my vital organs were shutting down. There was so much internalized failure to face, so many big questions I didn't have answers to. Wasn't this what I was supposed to want? Married at twenty-nine to a hot, successful, creative, beefy gentleman who loved the shit out of me and wanted a long life with me? How could I look such happiness in the face, turn, and run?

My family was gentle with Kip and me in our heartbreak. Nonetheless, I heard those old judgments bubble up from my subconscious and stare me in the face. *You run hot and cold. You're flighty. You eat men up and spit them out. You don't know what you want. And you don't even know what adult love—the "real" kind—looks like.*

It took a while for it to be over with Kip. Our lives tangled in so many places, and each knot had to be undone by hand. The unraveling of a life. Deciding what to do with the custom furniture we'd built to fit the space—he kept it. Who would deal with the dozens of framed pictures of us on the dining room collage wall?—I did. The blender we got as a wedding gift—we fought over it. Our shared dreams—we trashed them.

When the relationship was finally over, I was gutted, and I landed on my youngest sister Aba's couch for a few weeks. I spent my nights sobbing into a towel in the bathroom, hoping she wouldn't hear. She granted me the dignity of pretending she didn't. She had her own grief to bear; Kip had become like a brother to her.

There must be a word for the grief we experience over the life we thought we should have, events that never happened, stories that didn't have the happy ending. At every step in our path, some possibilities die behind us while others bloom before us, and in every transition, even the joyful ones, there is grief. From maiden to mother. Single to married. Unemployed to entrepreneur. The old you dies; a new one is born. The grief is ongoing, and never-ending.

It turns out, you can grieve both a dream and an untold future. One where the beloved brother-in-law is still alive, or you never left your home country. The one where we got that perfect job, and one where we pose, smiling, for the holiday card next to our chosen part- ner year after year, hair growing grayer, and children growing bigger.

It didn't matter, in the end, that married life wasn't *my* dream. It was *Cosmopolitan* magazine's. It belonged to the patriarchy and so- ciety. I was grieving the idea of a life that had never been mine, but still, I grieved. Cultural norms are like lead in our drinking water— you can be aware of their presence, but that doesn't make you any less sick.

For years, I blamed myself for the dissolution of our marriage. Kip was as good as they get, and I was the one who hadn't been strong enough to make it work. When I was offered a shot at the dream life, I was the one who had turned and fled down the freeway. The failure was mine, but the repercussions affected him deeply.

And yet now, more than fifteen years later, Kip and I no longer look like failure to me. We're still good friends. We still share a AAA account. He can still type the words to one of his little songs in a text, and I'll smile. He's as beautiful, genuine, and earnest as when we met, plus some gray hairs in his locs and a lot more sneakers. It's a joy watching the man he became after we split, even if that man isn't mine. He was never mine to keep, as I was not his.

The risk of loving anything is to lose it. Even when love follows the traditional romantic narrative of "till death do us part," eventually death arrives. It is painfully obvious and simple: love anyone, and one day your heart will break. Yet somehow humans choose to do it over and over again. Heartbreak itself is a death: the death of the relationship, the death of the person we are in the relationship, the death of a shared future. And with death comes grief. Grief is also the fertile soil from which we can be renewed.

That begs the question: When our hearts are broken open, what seedling of self can emerge more fortified in the aftermath? Because if a person could die from heartbreak, I would have died a hundred times by now. (Give or take.) And I would have also put myself back together stronger, richer, and indelibly marked by the price and payoffs of love.

In that moment when Kip held a ring glinting with promise in the freeway lights, my body was intelligent enough to know the truth of what I really wanted but could not admit. It told me to turn and run. It was only a matter of time before I was forced to accept that truth and learn to live with it. Many spend their lives fighting against what they know to be true, but most damning of all is when we fight against endings that are due to come, like death.

Using the keyless entry to Elena and Mike's modest home in a Beverly Hills–adjacent neighborhood in Los Angeles, I grab the notepad by the door. The tasks have been outlined clearly by Elena. My first task is to take off my shoes. Next, I am to wash my hands in the bathroom off the living room to avoid bringing bacteria or viruses to Mike. Because of ALS, his ability to cough and clear mucus is severely compromised, and a common virus like a cold or the flu could kill him. After washing my hands and doubling up with hand sanitizer, I am to make myself known by standing in the doorway of the bedroom until he acknowledges me and invites me in. If he isn't in the mood for a visitor, Elena warns, I'd know.

I met Elena three months before Mike died. She contacted me to provide additional respite support while she goes on an annual girls' trip with her best friends from college. Mike insisted that she go, even though she does not want to leave her beloved's side. My role is to visit for an hour each day, take stock of his disease and spirits, make sure the caregivers are doing their job, and to report back to Elena.

Mike and Elena are going it mostly alone. They have no children and moved to Los Angeles a year and a half after Mike's diagnosis. Since Elena quit her job to care for Mike and they barely have friends, their circle only consists of the hospice doctors, nurses, and certified nursing assistants (CNAs), some of whom will be present twenty-four hours a day during Elena's trip. To make herself feel better about leaving, Elena leaves a long list of instructions, including how to turn the television off. There are even instructions on how to compost egg shells—*grind them down first so they decompose quicker*. At the top of the legal notepad it says *DO NOT ASK HIM ABOUT YESTERDAY*.

I am familiar with ALS. My friend Richard's father died from the disease years ago. ALS causes the death of the neurons that control the voluntary muscles. Most people with ALS slowly lose the ability to walk, talk, use their limbs, swallow, and breathe. The erosion eats away at the body, making it increasingly difficult to perform the most basic functions of life. Caregiving for someone with ALS is a race to meet the emotional demands of each new loss, causing a veritable jungle gym of grief and ancillary losses.

Lying in an adjustable medical bed in their bedroom with the blinds closed, Mike invites me closer by tipping up his scruffy salt-and-pepper chin while keeping his eyes on the silent television.

"Should I open the blinds?" I whisper, trying to confirm he is aware of my presence without startling him.

He barely shakes his head no, still not looking my way.

I am relieved. The blinds aren't on my list, and Elena's detailed instructions on everything have put the fear of Moses into me. I cross the threshold into the bedroom but stand close to the doorway.

Vials of liquid medications, empty IV tubes, Kleenex, and a pestle and mortar for grinding pills are displayed on the nightstand. Mike's ability to project and communicate verbally are limited by the weakened muscles in his larynx, diaphragm, and throat. The television remote control lies just under his hand, ready to be deployed at any time.

He whispers, "What did she tell you about me?"

"Everything!" I respond with a laugh.

He chuckles weakly, still not looking at me. Then he cuts right to the chase. "She told you not to ask me about yesterday, right?"

I hesitate, unsure if saying yes would constitute a breach of confidence. Instead, I smile awkwardly, even though he isn't looking at me. This is my default facial expression when I don't know what to do, think, or say, insides boiling in social anxiety.

Mike continues, oblivious to my discomfort. "I know she did. Elena is worried every day." He takes a labored and audible breath. "She asks me to lift my fingers and marks how close I came to yesterday's mark. Like how you measure a kid against the wall in the kitchen every year." He draws another ragged breath. "I hate it. But I know she is just scared and so I do it." His eyes are fixed on the soundless television. "Do we have to do it while she is gone?"

I scan the list of instructions, flipping through four pages on the legal pad, plus the notes I made during my initial meeting with Elena. Despite her vigilance, Elena hadn't mentioned this private measuring ritual. I don't want to piss her off when she comes home, but I would have remembered something like that.

I respond tentatively. "No, I don't think so."

"Good." His eyes remain on the silent television, a news show in which talking heads gesticulate wildly at each other and vie for attention. Since Mike opened the door to talk about yesterday, I walk through it: "So, what about yesterday do you think she is afraid of?"

"She is scared that every day I am one day closer to dying than I was the day before," he says, staring blankly at the red-faced news anchors. Finally, he turns his head slowly to look at me. "We all are. But she can actually tell that I am getting closer when I can't do the things I used to anymore. I gave up being angry about today because of yesterday a long time ago, but my wife is doing it her way. Every day is like a brand-new day for her." With his weakened voice, I heard "Every day is like a brand-new death for her." He's not wrong either way. Each day is the death of the Mike from the day before. He's making his peace at a different pace than Elena is.

During our first meeting, Elena, formerly a bookkeeper with shoulder-length graying hair and red-framed drugstore readers, showed me the spreadsheets she'd made to chart every facet of Mike's care. Doctors, pharmacists, reactions, foods, timetables—you name it, Elena had a spreadsheet for it. Some part of me, I admit, shivered at the neatly tabbed rows. I've never met a spreadsheet I liked. But even though Elena was my total opposite in many ways, I spotted something too familiar to ignore behind those drugstore reading glasses.

I too had struggled for months, clinging to one dearly held belief at a time, in the face of a truth that felt just too big and too awful to accept. When my marriage with Kip dissolved, it didn't happen in a blinding flash. It was a series of small losses, and each day brought a new reckoning. I might not have used a spreadsheet, but you can bet that I also measured the distance between yesterday's truth and today's. Each day, and each loss, brought with it a new spasm of grief.

In truth, Elena's spreadsheets are an ingenious coping mechanism. She is controlling what she can. If she can't control how far Mike can stretch his fingers each day, she can at least keep a detailed log. This is how Elena is managing her grief, by doubling down on what she does so well: marking, measuring, recording. They are a yardstick to mark her husband's deterioration as well as the level of her daily loss.

Asking Mike about yesterday defeats Elena's efforts to stay in the present with his disease. So she doesn't ask; she measures. It might look rigid, but it works for her. And when caregivers find something that works for them so that they can keep taking care of the dying, everybody wins.

People with degenerative diseases such as Alzheimer's and multiple sclerosis and those who care for them often become reluctant experts in adaptability. In these conditions and many others, there is a gradual weakening and degeneration of the body, one system at a time. People who live with these diseases and those who care for them are forced to become masterful adapters. To adapt is central to the human experience. Humans are masters at navigating the unknown and adapting to new circumstances, even though we often do not give ourselves the credit. Change is the god that we *must* bow to.

Each new day that we get to wake up, we greet a reality that wages a war of attrition against our expectations. Life doesn't go the way we want. Duh. Ideas fail. People change their minds. Governments get overthrown. Babies won't nap. Psychedelic trips end with a potential for inpatient treatment. Our hearts get broken. We burn dinner. Tires go flat. Yet, we learn to adapt in the moment, even as we struggle and resist. Learning to adapt introduces us to the new self, time and time again. The new self is one we never imagined—someone who has integrated all that has come before.

When we arrive at this new place, we are able to say, "Today, I am here." Starting sentences and thoughts with the word *today* grounds us in the present. "Today, my husband can no longer walk." "Today, I can't grip my coffee cup." "Today, my best friend can't stomach her favorite meal." "Today, I am separated." "Today, my father is dead." Today is not without its grief.

I continue to visit Mike and Elena for the next three months until Mike dies. After our sticky beginning, we've grown close. During our visits when Elena turns her head or leaves the room Mike secretly lifts his finger for me and smiles weakly. It's become our inside language to signal that Elena is keeping up her ritual. She's never shared this private practice of hers with me and I've never revealed that I know. It endears me to her. I am also touched that Mike is allowing his wife to move at her own pace with his dying, as a part of her is dying with him. As expected, eventually he isn't able to lift his finger any more.

When Elena calls to tell me that Mike has been diagnosed with pneumonia—a common occurrence for people with late-stage ALS—we both know that the end is near, especially since Mike has chosen not to treat it. Over the phone, she recites everything the doctor has said and the changes she's made to her spreadsheets to include how many breaths he is taking a minute and how often he coughs. When the breaths slow considerably and Mike struggles to clear his airway, she sits with him until his respiratory function stops altogether. Mike is dead.

I visit with them later that day. Elena sits in the same chair she sat in during his illness with her laptop on her lap, but this time it is closed. The TV is off, and Mike is still in the bed, awaiting transport by the funeral home. She seems distant, in the shock of acute grief, the impossible having happened before her eyes. I gently take the laptop from her, set it down, and ask permission to take her hand. She lets me. Then she finally cries and I cry with her.

After Mike's death, Elena struggles to adapt to her own new normal of having no one aside from herself to care for. For almost two years, her entire life has been focused on Mike's care. She doesn't have any more spreadsheets to update, and nothing outside of herself to control. We talk on and off about the tasks to wrap up his affairs, but Elena handled most of them while he was living. She sorely misses his presence beside her at night, as she slept in a bed right next to his hospital bed. Less than a year after Mike's death, when all the chores are done, the hospital bed removed, his clothes given away and his sentimental items boxed, Elena dies of a heart attack. I believe she dies of a broken heart. Nothing left to live for.

In my work as a death doula, I journey with clients from their old self to their new self, even if their new self is the deathbed self. Understandably, people struggle to integrate their own impending mortality or the mortality of someone they love. To support them practically to ground in the now, I offer clients a practice I call "finding your feet." When I'm with someone focused on the past or worried about the future, I encourage them to join me in the present, with a simple reminder about their feet. The mind can travel. The body is always right here. By bringing attention to the feet and thus into the body, either by enjoying a warm foot bath or simply placing our bare feet firmly on the earth and wiggling our toes, we can invite ourselves into the moment that we can utter these life-affirming words of adaptability: "Today, I am here."

Kip was my first time learning what happens when you try to fight the truth you see in front of you. You wind up locked into an exhausting struggle against yourself, a struggle in which you can only ever lose. We must reckon with our truths daily. If only I could have learned this lesson just once. But like all of us, I would have to learn it again and again. Soon, I would start learning it with my so-called "career."

Chapter 9

Fighting Losing Battles

On my first day as a "real" lawyer at the Legal Aid Foundation of Los Angeles, where I'd been hired a few months after moving in with Kip, I stared at the little office with my name on it. The frosted-glass door said "Alua Arthur Attorney" in adhesive letters. I scratched at the corner of the *A* in *Attorney* to see if it could come off. When it gave a little, I breathed a sigh of relief. The nameplate wasn't permanent. I smoothed it back into place so no one would notice, putting off for another day my truth that I did not want to be a lawyer. This denial wore me down sneakily for almost nine years until only that truth remained. Then it had to be faced. But my body already knew.

My first role was as a staff attorney in the government benefits unit, where I advocated for people who'd lost access to benefits to which they were entitled—food stamps, cash aid, health coverage. This was my first full-time office job, excluding summer internships, and I was embarrassed to discover how much I struggled with a regular schedule. Legal Aid offices didn't even have the same high-performance, working-at-all-hours culture of big law firms. Everyone was expected to be in by nine, but few people worked past five. It was a simple arrangement, and I didn't know anyone else who chafed against it.

But it felt restrictive and I fidgeted just thinking about it. What if I was cranky in the morning and needed some time to remember how to talk to people again? Mornings have always been hard for me. Every Christmas for about six years, my parents ignored my request for a guitar and bought me watches instead, all of which piled up, unworn, on the dresser. They tried to get me to care about time but I don't. It's an illusion. Being on time has never been my forte, let alone before 11 A.M.

After only a year working in government benefits, I grew restless. Seeing the inner workings of the government disgusted me. Budgets got cut, benefits were diminished, and people continued to suffer despite the country's tremendous wealth. Clients, who were mostly Black and Brown, returned again and again after getting kicked off of their benefits, all because they had accidentally made just a little bit of money over the cap. Applicants would have to wait in obscene lines at the government offices to turn in paperwork, all just to keep a measly $221 in cash aid a month for a single able-bodied person. That doesn't buy shit in Los Angeles. The government doesn't care about poor people, and I got tired of going up against the bureaucracy, which is designed to keep them that way.

Frustrated and beat down over not being able to make more of an impact, I sought a lateral transfer to the family law unit, doing domestic violence work. Working out of the courthouse a couple days a week, we'd have a few hours to get restraining orders, file divorces or custody requests, and get our clients into shelters away from their abusers. The constant motion, the urgency, and the ever-changing legal landscape quelled my boredom a bit, and I got to work with friends like Patima Komolamit, who ran the Center for the Pacific Asian Family's secret domestic violence shelter. Standing about five-three, with curly purple hair tied up with bejeweled chopsticks, Patima and I often drank wine over a mountain of cheese and carbohydrates, eating away our frustrations at the system.

But despite the camaraderie, the work got stagnant. Aside from the action in the courtroom, the day-to-day work of a family lawyer is surprisingly pretty dull. Paperwork. Client meetings. More paperwork. Court. Paperwork. I felt myself growing numb, and then I'd curse myself for that numbness. Clients kept coming back seeking protection from the same abusers. They told me repeated stories of their partners locking them in or out of the house, putting bleach in their food, forcibly cutting their hair, rape, withholding money, using children as pawns in their desperate and pathetic ploys for power, and using them as punching bags. Even with the knowledge that it can take about seven attempts to leave a domestic abuse situation, it was hard for me to see an end to the cycles of violence from where I sat.

I felt powerless and was burning out. I'd cry in the bathrooms in between hearings when the situation was desperate, hoping my clients weren't in there too. I'd been practicing law for four years, but I could already sense something in me was dying. My heart felt like concrete. I was losing myself, my sensitivity, and my faith in humanity.

With mounting fear—why wasn't this working? What was wrong?—I switched roles *again* within Legal Aid, this time to go to the community economic development unit. Cutting my hours made me a part-time employee, a perverse decision for any lawyer. For a single woman with no high-earning partner or children to care for, it was practically unheard-of. It was pretty apparent that only those with family money or rich husbands were allowed the full freedom to determine the conditions under which they worked. But I was already used to being broke. I just wanted to be free.

I convinced myself that working twenty-one hours a week with community leaders starting charter schools in low-income neighbor-hoods in L.A. would scratch the eternal itch, the one that had been with me for as long as I could remember: the fear of boredom. Com-placency. The dulling of my inner light, the dimming of my natural curiosity. I'd dismantled anything I could get my hands on as a kid to stave it off. Now, it seemed like I could not stop myself from doing the same thing to my Legal Aid career.

Looking back at this time, I can already see a woman who was losing a battle. I could have peeled my name completely off the door and never looked back. Just like with Kip, my feet were already itching to run away, but I took that urge to run away and steered myself, over and over, right back into my work, telling myself that this was what I was supposed to do. Every transfer I made at Legal Aid was an evasive maneuver. I was running toward justice, yes. But I was also running away from myself.

Unsure how to fight against this creeping rot, I'd ride my bike nine miles to work, with headphones in my ears, weaving through traffic in L.A. singing at the top of my lungs and feeling the sun on my skin. Swimming in endorphins was the only way I could counteract the dread. I'd arrive sweaty, breathless, and always late, freshen up in the ladies' room, change out of denim shorts and into my "lawyer clothes" in my office, and get to work. Since I was part-time, some weeks I'd work a lot of hours to free my schedule to take time off and travel when I wanted.

For almost four more years, this schedule staved off the existential dread long enough for me to feel some measure of balance. Sure, I wasn't happy in my job, but there were other things in life—right? This dead corner inside of me would surely heal on its own.

To satiate my roving mind and keep my creative self alive, I began a freelance photography business, shooting destination weddings, stills for international documentaries, and general street photography. I carried a camera everywhere with me, even in my bike bag on the way to work in case I saw something that helped me see the beauty in humankind.

My other go-to boredom cure, then as now, was travel. Boredom functions in the mind like pain functions in the body. It alerts you that something is up. But I looked away. Whenever work got dull or I was going through a romantic breakup, rather than sit with the discomfort of being with myself and making the changes necessary, I'd run off. Some people get bangs; I booked solo international journeys.

My travels were not glamorous. Hostels, budget train cars, and multiple layovers resulted in long travel days, which was all I could afford on my part-time Legal Aid lawyer's budget. But that was okay—it kept me distracted, and also kept my racing mind busy. I was looking for something to save me from myself during this period, yet it seemed that wherever I went, there I was. As my malaise grew, the world seemed to shrink. There was no place I could go, no adventure grand enough where I wouldn't step off the plane and find it waiting for me.

I hoped that perhaps I'd fall in love with a man in Caracas, Venezuela, and he would give me a new life, since my last new life kept stubbornly reverting back to the old one. So I tried. But Marcos was twenty-three years old and still lived with his mom. I came home to my boring and unfulfilled life in Los Angeles.

I traveled anywhere that could hold my interest, which was quite a challenge for an attention span like mine. I feel most alive when I am curious, and it's impossible for me not to be curious when I'm traveling. I wanted to see how other people outside of the dominant Western culture lived, what they loved, how they showered, what shoes they wore, how the moon looked from their longitude and latitude, how heavy their coins were in my pocket. A voyeur in someone else's country, and in someone else's life—anyone's but my own. What foods did they eat out of bowls and what social etiquettes did they follow? Perhaps they had answers to the big questions in life that I was lacking. Perhaps, on one of these trips, I would finally find the cure to whatever seemed to be slowly killing me inside.

Most of my travel was with just a backpack, exploring developing countries on a dime and tasting random and unfamiliar street food, salmonella be damned. I'd settle on a random destination from the airport, exchange some money, and call my parents to let them know I was safe and promise to be in touch in a few days. When I was firmly planted in this new place, I talked to strangers in bars and on the street, to learn what to do and where to go next. Using this method, I sunbathed naked on private beaches on Isla de Margarita, Venezuela; sipped Assam tea in Myanmar; discovered the best jazz spot in Johannesburg; and rode the entire island of Barbados on the back of a motorcycle driven by a handsome man named Davy Jones.

I've done some foolish shit too. All were desperate grasps at an experience in an effort to feel something. *Anything*.

I came down from a mountain hike in Honduras on hands and knees, trembling, because I was terrified of the switchbacks. I went skydiving in New Zealand to kick my crippling fear of heights up a notch to see if I could cure it. It made my fear *much* worse. I've taken dodgy buses to strange locations with no place to sleep once there, to meet up with brand-new "friends" I've just met, without so much as a phone number or a last name to find them. Once, in Fiji, I stayed up all night drinking hallucinogenic kava root with the staff at the resort and set out alone in a kayak the following morning to reach the Blue Lagoon. My body was exhausted, the sun bearing down relentlessly, and by the time I made it, ragged and gasping, I had no energy for the return trip. I staggered onto the beach, arms limp, and slept, rousing myself to make it back before dark.

Unsurprisingly, my spontaneity sometimes landed me in dubious circumstances. I was held by authorities in Mexico on my way back to Los Angeles because they couldn't validate the authenticity of my green card—or so they said. In India, I was mobbed by followers of the goddess Kali—dark skin, hair like rope, a garland of men's severed heads around her neck. Not totally inaccurate, but I thought I hid my romantic past better than that. They touched my hair, and grabbed at my clothing. In my travels, particularly to places where not a lot of Black people travel, I grew accustomed to feeling like the constant object of both fascination and suspicion—tall, dark, female, and traveling alone apparently wasn't a common sight. But for a moment at the Golden Temple in Amritsar, India, I imagined, *This is what it's like to be Britney Spears*—caged by attention, every move dissected and made fodder for the delight of the public. Brutal. But I still preferred it to being at home.

Another time, I got trapped deep in an alley in the busy and colorful open-air Khan el-Khalili market in Cairo, surrounded by ominous-looking men near an ATM. They stared at me like they'd seen a four-course meal and exchanged looks. My intuition told me they were interested in my body and not my money. One of them grabbed me, but I ran and kicked my way out of the alley until I was in the light of the market again.

After the scare in the alley, I was eager to get back to the safety of the hotel before my flight home the next day. I'd been fascinated by the history in Egypt; looking at a wig worn by Cleopatra thousands of years ago put my piddly thirty-two years of life in some much-needed perspective. Who cared that I was starting to hate my job and couldn't get dressed when there had been billions of people who had already lived and died, each with their own struggles and wigs? So I gathered myself, negotiated a fare with a taxi driver, and plopped down in the relative safety of his cab. As we made our way back to my hotel, the driver and I sat in traffic like a parking lot, inhaling exhaust fumes and making small talk.

"You from Africa?" he asked, eyeing me in the rearview mirror. This question had previously been a source of ire, as I'd been in a few heated conversations with Egyptians who didn't call themselves African. They insisted they were Middle Eastern. As far as I know from the maps, Egypt sits on the mighty continent of Africa.

"Yes, I am from Ghana," I replied, hoping to not have a redo of the same conversation.

"You sound like American."

"I was raised mostly in the States. I live in California." Because of his efforts, I made an attempt to soften. I was mistaken.

After an ominous silence, he sighed loudly and spat out the window, murmuring some words in Arabic. "Listen, lady. Too much traffic now. You pay more, okay?" He looked at me, annoyed, over his shoulder.

Ah shit. Not now.

He continued. "You have money. You leave Africa and you go to

America, you have money." This was a common tactic I was used to. After agreeing on a price, a driver takes you into traffic, then asks for more money because it is "farther" than they thought. After my poor negotiating at the market that afternoon, where I overpaid for an aluminum hookah thinking it was brass, I didn't want to be taken advantage of again. Now, it felt like he wanted to extort me because of my West African face and American accent. I refused.

Gesturing wildly at the cars in front of him, he spewed a bunch of words in Arabic and spit out the window again. "You don't understand anything. You are stupid. You Africans are so stupid. I know why they made you slaves! Because you are stupid! Stupid! STUPID!" His hands flew, emphasizing his words, ash flying around the car as he grew more enraged with each hateful word. Stunned and scared of his escalating temper, I gathered my bags of goodies from the market in a hurry, got out of the cab, and slammed the door behind me. He continued yelling out the window as I maneuvered through multiple lanes of traffic on foot to make it to the sidewalk. It was dusk and the women had started slowly disappearing from the streets. I was alone in the middle of Cairo.

A man working at a kiosk who had heard the commotion motioned me inside his store. Using his young son as a translator, he apologized on behalf of the taxi driver and explained that I was only one long block away from the hotel. The taxi driver had tried to circle around to get a higher fare. Since the women had left the streets, the store owner put his son in charge and walked me back to my hotel. I wanted to hug him but it would have gone against social norms so I teared up in gratitude instead. I didn't leave the hotel again until my ride to the airport.

Nonetheless, even these brushes with real danger weren't enough to put me off travel. Once the danger faded, there was even something addictive in the fear itself. Abandoned, running away from attackers, drinking narcotics—at least I wasn't bored.

I kept seeking and going on to the next adventure, the next bizarre encounter, the next laugh. Yak rides in Cambodia, four trips to Carnaval in Salvador, Brazil, overripe mangosteen in Laos, dawn hikes on broken steps to Adam's Peak in Sri Lanka—the more foreign, the better.

Returning home once more, I'd take my time unpacking, smelling the black plastic bags of my purchases, hoping they would transport me out of my apartment and back to wherever I just came from. Soon enough, smells faded, as did the buzz of the adventure, and the stories I told about my trip over brunch got old. Once the peaks faded, it was clear nothing had changed. All that remained were passport stamps and my yearning.

I distracted and distracted and distracted myself. I ran away from my pain of not knowing why I was doing the work I was doing, trying to patch together a life that felt good. Why was I fighting so hard to remain engaged in the life I'd built for myself? Why did no one else around me seem to be struggling like I was? How did they have it figured out?

It looks like Jordan has it figured out. At twenty-seven years old and a working actor, complete with Hallmark-movie romantic lead looks and action figure–size, he has no reason to believe that he is near the end of his life. He is not sick. Yet he has an intense fear of death. It expresses itself via fear of catastrophies, often very unlikely ones— tsunamis, the bubonic plague, atomic bombs, even raining swords. The thoughts arise seemingly out of nowhere and cause a stress response in his body, crippling him mentally. They have begun to interfere with his life. Jordan has lost job opportunities where he was asked to perform action sequences, and he lost a girlfriend who loved going to the beach. His fear of tsunamis kept him away from the water.

Jordan addresses most of his anxieties through talk therapy, along with a heavy dose of magical thinking—*If I stop at every single stop sign for exactly six seconds, I won't get in a car accident. If I blink three times before I turn on the light, I will not have an aneurysm.* He's taken ayahuasca journeys, used other psychedelics, and is on a daily cocktail of anti-anxiety medications. Still, vestiges of fear remain within his body. He wants to get to the bottom of it, or at least become more familiar with its roots and I tend to believe that anxieties and fears derive from a fear of death. I've never felt the exact fears that Jordan feels, but I too have clocked many hours running away from worries that only grew larger the harder I ran. I remember how awful it feels. I agree to help.

Jordan feels that confronting his death directly could support him. I ask him to talk to his psychiatrist first about a service I offer called death meditation. The psychiatrist agrees to talk to me directly about the process. I explain that under my watchful eye, I would move with Jordan through a meditation called the Nine Contemplations on Death, written by Atisha, an eleventh-century Buddhist scholar and developed further by roshi Joan Halifax and Larry Rosenberg, with my additional spin on it. These contemplations help us explore the inevitability of death and notice what is important in light of our mortality. The meditation then moves into envisioning the body's eventual end. I ask meditators to pay attention to which contemplations or thoughts make them uncomfortable.

The psychiatrist is curious about the experience and compares the meditation to exposure therapy. I don't disagree but believe it to be far gentler than jumping out of a plane at twenty thousand feet to cure a fear of heights like I tried in New Zealand. After having done dozens of these meditation sessions with individual clients and several in a group setting, I'm certain that it could be useful for Jordan. We schedule his death meditation session with the approval of his psychiatrist.

As part of the prep for the session, Jordan and I discuss his major fears around death. In order to help him imagine his death in a non-triggering manner, we talk through his most ideal death, which he is able to do with surprising ease. He can imagine dying in his bed, where he falls asleep and never wakes up again. It is a pretty basic ideal death, considering raining swords are an option in his brain.

For the meditation session, I try to re-create Jordan's ideal death by setting up his bedroom in his apartment in Echo Park, across the street from the lake. His bedroom is already softly lit with lamps with linen lampshades, so I add some tea lights around his bed, which sits low to the ground. I ask his permission to light some candles and then ask him to trust me enough to lie on the bed in the middle of the tea lights on the floor, as he also fears fires. Trust is critical if I'm going to lead him to his death, even if only in his mind.

Jordan takes a sip of water from the glass on his nightstand, also placed there to calm his fear of fires. He is dressed in pajamas to mimic dying while asleep. Cautiously, he lies down in the center of the bed and closes his eyes. I cover him with a blue and brown quilt made by his grandma that he still uses to quell his anxiety. It barely reaches his knees. On top of that I place a weighted blanket to soothe him further. The meditation isn't dangerous, and I'll be watching the entire time. But I want Jordan to feel safe. I tell him that he is.

We begin by breathing deeply together, then walk through an exercise to relax his muscles and coax his body toward calmness. I slowly begin to guide Jordan through the meditation. We start with the first contemplation of dying: Death is inevitable. On the in breath, I ask him to repeat to himself, "Death is inevitable." On the out breath, "I too will die." On the second contemplation, I ask Jordan to breathe in that his life span is ever decreasing, and on his out breath to contemplate if he never took another breath. The third contemplation is "Death comes whether or not I am prepared," breathing in with awareness of all he has yet to complete, and breathing out his attachment to completing any of it. On the fourth, we consider that our life spans are not fixed. On Jordan's in breath, I ask him to bring awareness to the tremendous mystery of the end of his life and on his out breath, release attachment to knowing.

When I get to the fifth contemplation of dying—Death Has Many Causes—Jordan's body begins to squirm around when he had previously been still and immersed. A little concerned, I stop the meditation to ask if he is okay. Jordan sits straight up, wild-eyed, but says he wants to keep going. His voice is tight and he seems uncomfortable, but eager. I've learned to trust people with their healing, so I agree to keep going. Even though he's terrified, he wants to move forward. I am inspired by his courage.

Jordan lies back down, and I tuck him into his grandma's quilt and weighted blanket again. We haven't even started the most difficult part. We take a few more deep breaths to ground ourselves back in the experience and through the remaining contemplations: my body is fragile and vulnerable, my material resources will be of no use to me, my loved ones cannot save me, and my own body cannot help me when death comes. When I wrap up the ninth contemplation and check in again with Jordan, he wiggles his hand free of the blanket to give me a strong thumbs-up. Then he opens one eye to make sure the bed isn't on fire.

In the next section of the meditation, I walk Jordan through a process that asks him to visualize his body shutting down, going through the organs of the body methodically. We imagine them losing oxygen-rich blood and nutrients, and eventually dying. Jordan's eyes flutter slightly, but he keeps breathing evenly with his eyes closed. I continue.

Since Jordan has suggested that he wants to be buried and not cremated (he cannot imagine his body on fire), we consider his body's decomposition and the decaying bones, which eventually become dust. Jordan's breathing stays steady and light: gentle inhalations and exhalations of air. The meditation is going well.

Next, I ask Jordan to imagine life continuing in his absence—his family members, friends, loved ones, and strangers carrying on their activities of living without him. His breathing gets deeper but stays steady. At the conclusion of the meditation, I invite Jordan back into his body and his room, ask him to move his arms, contract and release his muscles, stretch his legs toward the wall and his arms overhead. The vital life force is swirling within him. Not yet dead.

Jordan's eyes are wet, and he looks like he has emerged from a deep sleep. I ask him to rotate his ankles and wrists, to again flex and relax the muscles in his legs and arms, and wiggle his body like a popcorn shrimp in oil. With a chuckle, he says that he is hungry and could go for some shrimp right now, which I take as a sign that he's fully back.

He tells me that as he imagined his body's end, he was at peace. He felt sad that he was no longer around but had no resistance to his death. The parts that made him most uncomfortable were the parts about dying: the reality that the body is vulnerable and death has many causes. His fear is rooted in the process of dying and the possible pain. Jordan's fear of pain ballooned into a fear of any event that might cause a painful death, which led to his fixation on catastrophic events he could not control, like tsunamis, instead of old age or disease. This is not unusual. Jordan doesn't fear death itself. Just dying.

I acknowledge Jordan's discomfort and offer some information around how we die because he says it will support him. For years Jordan has been staying out of situations that could cause his death. He avoided amusement parks because he could fall off a roller coaster. He got anxious driving over bridges because the infrastructure could collapse. He wouldn't get a motorcycle, even though he longed to own one, to ride it up the Pacific Coast Highway, his ex-girlfriend on the back. But he lost the girlfriend and never dared to buy the bike.

While motorcycle accidents sometimes do happen, the vast majority of motorcycle owners die as a result of disease. *Most* of us die as a result of disease. According to the Centers for Disease Control and Prevention's National Vital Statistics Report on mortality, only about 6 percent of people in the United States die as a result of an unintentional injury or accident.

Avoiding pain has been a primary motivator in Jordan's life. He notices it as a theme. What we fear about death often is also present in our lives. Unconsciously, he's been running away from pain and the possibility of dying rather than toward pleasure. In taking all these steps to avoid death, he's also been putting off his life: the one where he is a successful action star doing stunts, going on adventures, and in love. *Don't do the stunts, you will get hurt and die. Don't open your heart, it will break. Don't love, you will grieve. Don't live, you will die.*

This is a common tactic to escape our deep-seated fear of death—avoid avoid avoid. But to be alive on this planet is to be subject to millions of causes and conditions that could result in our death, even though disease of the body is the most common. There are as many different ways to die as there are stars in the sky: accidents, disease, or so-called acts of God, like natural disasters, earthquakes, and storms. Death could come at the hand of another or a slip down the stairs. So often when we hear that someone has died, one of the very first questions we ask is "How?" It is deeply ingrained within us to want to understand the circumstances that lead to a death, to either blame the person for their carelessness or to sympathize with their misfortune. We victim-shame people who die rather than just accept death as a normal and natural cycle of life that they have no control over, except for when they choose it. Perhaps we feel as though we can exercise some control over the "how" (if you weren't so careless you wouldn't have died), but never the "what" (you're gonna die anyway).

Still, avoidance is not the solution. When we don't do the things we want to do out of fear that they could kill us or hurt us, we rob ourselves of the gift of life. How avoidance shows up varies from person to person, and it can be sneaky. It can even camouflage itself as virtuous behavior such as perfectionism, workaholism, obsessive cleaning, or adventurous travel. And then there are the more destructive examples, like death denial, all forms of addiction, and debilitating procrastination. In all these instances, we are avoiding facing something and stuffing it down with something else. But what I've seen in my work and experienced in my life is that avoidance only works for so long, until we must show up for whatever we are avoiding. Not showing up for it doesn't make it go away. One way or another, it will be waiting for you.

Chapter 10

Hexagon-Shaped Peg

Sometimes, we're blessed with unexpected guardian figures in life. Here you are, running away from some all-consuming truth, and then, life serves you up someone who narrows their eyes at you and names the very thing you're avoiding so desperately. Usually, they are tough but compassionate. They come to you in the spirit of guidance, not shame. They are doula figures, patrolling self-denial's wilderness to point you, gently but firmly, toward the path of truth of self.

For me, this person was Silvia Argueta.

I vividly remember when I first met Silvia. A senior attorney at the Legal Aid Foundation of Los Angeles, a first-generation Guatemalan American, and the first person in her family to go to college, let alone become a lawyer, she was a force in her own right, and I was drawn to her immediately. Immigrant sees immigrant, even though at her height—four feet eleven inches, never rounding up to five feet because that would be a lie—I often only saw the top of her head. During my tortured tenure, she became a mentor and close friend.

When Silvia's father died, I attended his funeral. When she spoke to a medium afterward, hoping to reach him, the woman asked to speak to the tall smiley Black woman in the office. Meaning me. The next day, Silvia knocked on my door and told me about the medium's request as if she were relaying a sandwich order. I was spooked, but

I talked to the medium anyway. (Apparently, my grandma I'd never met wanted to say hi.)

When I was repeatedly frustrated by the inequities of the benefits programs, Silvia listened to me bitch, my tears brimming about the injustice of it all. But in that first meeting, she got right to the point with me.

"Why are you a lawyer?"

The question unnerved me. It was so direct and, in this setting, so obvious, though I hadn't thought about it since my law school application essays—and even then, I bullshitted. "Well, um. . . ." I sniffled, fiddling with the rings on my hands, trying to conjure up something to appease this firecracker. "I want to impact justice somehow and help people and be there when people most need someone there and . . ." I trailed off, hoping I was convincing her. But I'm a terrible liar. All of this was true, but it didn't explain why I'd chosen the practice of law.

I was too embarrassed to tell her that I was a lawyer because I had been a "gifted" child expected to do big things with her life, and being a lawyer sounded good, and I wanted to make my family proud.

I couldn't tell her that I had not been brave enough to stop and understand what I wanted, and that despite the tremendous amount of work that law school and the bar exam had been, I had just taken the path of least resistance. It sounded silly even to me—when "the path of least resistance" involves putting yourself through the torture of law school and the agony of passing the California Bar Exam, with its pass rate of around 34 percent, you know you're running away from *something*.

I couldn't dare tell Silvia that I longed for a different life, which I was afraid to even visualize, and that I felt this life receding further from me every day. I didn't need to. Silvia saw my deep sensitivity, my difficulty with the nature of the work, and my quirky style. I was trying to fit a hexagon-shaped peg into a lawyer-sized hole, and Silvia saw right through me.

I think she was the only one. Everyone else in the office bought into my lawyer performance, which was a gift, because the good Lord knows I spent enough time and money trying to convince them. Throughout my nine years at Legal Aid, I shopped like I was stocking a store. In the months between travel adventures and boyfriends, when I felt the desperation mounting and I knew I wouldn't be able to get away, not even for a three-day weekend, one of my only remaining tricks was to buy new clothes.

However, this was a particularly bleak form of retail therapy, because I only bought drab "lawyer" clothes, trying to fit in. No orange Alexander McQueen ball gown skirts, no mudcloth capes from Accra. Instead, I bought heather-gray wool suits and pinstripe pantsuits, pencil skirts (not too tight as to show my ass), and periwinkle button-down dress shirts (not buttoned so high I'd look like a Pilgrim). Embellished belts, colored shoes, headbands, and accessories for the tiniest little drip.

Each day I'd put on an outfit and look at myself in the mirror, squinting to see from the perspective of my clients. As a young Black woman (who looked even younger given my high cheekbones and melanin), I had to try harder to be taken seriously by my clients, coworkers, opposing counsel, and judges. Would they respect me in this outfit? Did I look like a lawyer with gold jewelry hanging out of every visible orifice? What if I put on glasses? The practice of law is still an old white boys' club, and I did not want to present myself in a way that would be a hindrance to my clients. Did I look the part I was trying to play?

Clearly not to Silvia.

The clothes fit my body, which was losing weight because of all the bike riding and waning appetite. But they didn't fit *me*. My appearance is the message I am conveying about who I am. As the child of a model and designer, fashion sense is in my DNA. My mom touted her vanity and reinforced the idea that we can dress to help us cultivate joy. "Look good, feel good," my mom would tell us. I flood my body with dopamine through bright colors, soft fabrics, flowy silhouettes. When I put on *the* dress, I twirl by instinct. Despite the admonitions not to, humans judge books by their cover all the time, and I want mine to be as accurate as possible.

Each day is a chance to put together a look that is a reflection of my inner being, and when the outer shell no longer feels reflective of the inner self, I start to feel itchy, constrained. You can dismiss the importance of fashion, if you want. But clothes, to me, are freedom. They are expression and art. Above all, I want freedom to change: my mind, my heart, my clothes, my profession, my choices. When a style becomes constraining, all you have to do is look in the mirror and change it.

Some mornings, I would eye my favorite yellow chiffon tutu skirt but would talk myself out of wearing it to work. It wasn't "professional" enough. I'd take off my multicolored nail polish to present at board meetings and pull my locs back in a low ponytail for court. Each time I changed outfits because of fear that I didn't look the part, I traded a small piece of my authenticity to conform to a life I'd convinced myself I was supposed to want. I was trying to dress a zebra up as a horse.

I've always felt like a zebra, no matter where I was. Black in America, African with Black people, American in Ghana. The youngest student in community college math classes. The fat cheerleader, the vegetarian in my family, the girl with the short hair when everyone was wearing theirs long, who blurted out things that didn't make sense to other people and laughed at the joke in my head at inappropriate times. No matter where I went in this world, I didn't fit in. And the harder I tried to, the more I stuck out.

During a meeting at Legal Aid I referred to Twitter users as twats. I wasn't trying to be crude; I thought that was the right name. It made melodic sense. People who tweet are twats. Right? Wrong. The meeting didn't so much stop as crash land so the other attorneys could explain my error. I burned in my seat and they struck the conversation from the minutes. I didn't know it was a "bad word." English isn't my first language!

For the next eight years, as I switched practice groups, stifled myself, and continued to grow more discontented, Silvia would persistently ask me the question again: "Why are you a lawyer?" Each time I'd bullshit a new version of the same answer. But I was unconvincing. I was good with clients, but shit at the nuts and bolts of the job. I was (and am) disorganized—my papers were sprawled all over my desk, with crucial forms buried inside the mountain. I was temperamentally unsuited to debating the finer legal points. I was more interested in what was *right* rather than what was legal, which makes an excellent philosopher but a terrible lawyer.

I wanted to hold my clients' hands, tell their stories, cry with them, and love them into better situations for themselves. I wanted to talk about life, healing, and art. I'd work myself into a tizzy because of how ineffective the laws were and would drink a bottle of wine to numb myself after work. Silvia stuck with me, trying to help me find a position within Legal Aid that fit. She didn't nag. She trusted me with my life.

I didn't trust myself, though. I knew, deep down, something was wrong. I was wearing someone else's clothes, feeling like I was wearing someone else's skin. I had a wardrobe that didn't look like me. A career I'd backed myself into. Lies I told myself. A life that didn't even feel like mine.

One saving grace of this job was that it looked good on the outside. The other was that I only had to don the mask part-time. The rest of the time, I had the freedom to be me. For a while it was worth it to trade my authenticity for twenty-one hours a week. But year after year of smothering myself introduced an insidious ache I couldn't shake. It permeated my being.

I could barely recognize myself in the mirror. Whenever I pulled my locs back or fixed my button-down shirt, I saw an emptiness lurking behind my eyes, the same one I felt spreading through my body whenever I modulated my voice or suppressed my style at work. It was starting to suck away at my bone marrow—at my very essence.

Before long, my wardrobe started changing naturally. I veered toward grays and blacks. The colors faded. So did the effort. So did the spark of life within me. I thought I was doing what it took to survive, but in truth I was slowly killing myself. Shrinking my joy, murdering my own light. And for what? For a life I didn't buy into. It was like I was holding a pillow over my own face, waiting for myself to stop struggling.

I meet Ken shortly after hanging out my death doula shingle. His family found me to help get a power of attorney so they can manage his small business for him while he is dying in the hospital. I'm a little resistant to doing this, as I want to keep any legal work as far from my death work as possible, but I need clients. And I've got the skills. Death work requires that we bring our whole selves to the bedside, so I bring my legal skills this time too, even though I'd like to leave them far behind.

Ken owns a vintage clothing store in L.A. At fifty-seven, pancreatic cancer has worn his body down quickly. When I meet him in his hospital room, he is pallid, with downy baby hair from chemo, soft green eyes sunk deep in his skull, and naked bones visible in his wrist. When he was healthy, Ken—white, assigned male at birth, and using *he/him* pronouns—frequently wore skirts, blouses, stockings, heels, makeup, and tiaras. Today, he wears a standard-issue white-and-blue faded hospital gown—no eyeshadow, liner, blush, tiara, or lipstick. His family has never approved of his outfits, and in his illness, he's stopped trying. In illness, even the most fabulous of us revert to sweatpants and pajamas.

As Ken signs the power of attorney in front of a notary in his hospital bed, he seems defeated. I notice the fading flicks of green glitter nail polish and ask him about it when his sister leaves the room.

"I prefer my nails painted but 'they' don't like it." He gestures widely but weakly at the empty room, as though it held a full audience. I look around. Sometimes clients talk to people who I cannot see at the end of life and it is unclear if the dead are meeting the dying or if these are hallucinations that bubble up from the subconscious as the mind prepares itself for death. "Who in particular are you referring to?" I ask cautiously.

"They. My sister. My aunt. My dad. My nephew."

"Okay," I say, breathing a sigh of relief. I do not want to see dead people today. "When's the last time you painted them?" I ask.

"It's been a couple of months now. They asked me to stop, saying it would be confusing for other members of our biological family who have come to help out or visit. Nevermind that my chosen family has been here all along and they are just fine with it."

"Is that okay with you?"

"I'll do it for them when I am living. But if it were up to me, when they put me in the incinerator, I want blue nails with purple sparkle on them."

Ken's admission stirs something in me. I've spent years toning down my nail colors for others—for judges, opposing counsel, and summer law internships. If anyone ever needs a champion for the right to nail art in death or in life, they've got it in me.

"We can do that!" I say with a big smile.

Ken looks at me with such surprise I wonder if I misheard him. "You were serious about wanting glitter nails when you're cremated, weren't you?"

"I wasn't. But if you can do it, I am." His flat demeanor while discussing the power of attorney is changing.

"If you want it, I'll do my best to make that happen. What about your clothes?"

"I would rather wear a vintage gold pleated skirt with a pink leotard, but I'll wear a suit as long as it's not black. It pains me to think of that beautiful skirt being burned when I am cremated."

"Are you sure?" I press on, noticing that he is coming to life again talking about clothing. "If you want to wear the skirt, we can make that happen too."

Ken ponders this question from his hospital bed as he looks past the eggshell-colored walls with a stock ocean painting hanging near the window and out the eighth-floor window. From the length of his silence, it is clear he is considering it seriously.

He sighs. "I'm just trying to make it through these last days or weeks or months without pissing anyone off. I don't have it in me to fight for that."

"Well, I do!" I've got endless energy for battles for what I think is just, especially when it comes to the wishes of the dying. I quickly review the power of attorney Ken has just signed and I'm relieved we limited it to his business and financial decisions. Realistically, however, his family is still his next of kin, which means they will have the right to decide what he wears at his funeral and for the cremation, unless he makes clear plans himself or grants that right to someone else.

I see this all the time. Even when signing paperwork about what happens to their body after death, people often don't state outright what they want, leaving confusion for the surviving grieving family. The excuse is that they will be dead anyway, but that leaves the decision-making to their devastated circle of support. Ken knows all this but, understandably, can't be bothered. His funeral has been planned by his family, and he's fine with the fact that it will be held in a church. "I'll probably go up in flames as soon as they roll me in," he says dryly, gesturing heavenward. "It will save money on the cremation."

But I want to know more about what Ken *wants*, not just what he'll accept.

Since Ken loves clothing and seems to have ease talking about his death, we chat about funeral attire. Like me, he is tickled that people with breasts are often buried with a bra and that "burial shoes" exist.

We share a giggle about the modesty of the deceased. I tell Ken I can advocate for him with his family members if it's important to him. I inquire about the most sympathetic person to talk to. Maybe if they are swayed, the rest of the family will follow suit.

"Maybe my niece. But listen, it's not important to me that I wear my gold skirt in the coffin. I just want my nail polish." He sounds defeated again. I pause for a moment. While I'm familiar with stifled style, I can't fathom the pain of not being able to be fully expressed in my body. But that was me. Rather than continue to fight for what I would do, I back off and listen to my client. Just as I learned from my days working in legal services helping Tash that you can't live a client's life for them, I know now that neither can you die their death.

"Okay," I say. "Then I'm going to do my best to make sure you have blue and purple glitter nail polish in your coffin. Would that make you happy?"

Ken cracks a tired smile. "That would make me jubilant. I thought you came for my bank account, not for my nails."

By the time I leave, I am fired up for a battle with Ken's biological family over his fingernails. It's early days in my work as a death doula, but I know for sure that my role is to advocate for the dying person first.

Luckily, it only takes a couple of phone calls. Ken's niece is moved by her uncle's request and talks to her family members with my coaching. I suggest she tell them of the compromise he is willing to make to keep them happy. They capitulate under the stipulation that his hands are by his sides in the coffin rather than crossed over his chest, so they wouldn't be seen during the open casket viewing. It is another small slight against being seen in his glory, but Ken is satisfied, and thus so am I. I call the funeral home to see if it would be possible and they agree.

Ken dies about two weeks after our conversation about his nails. His body doesn't combust in the church and he goes triumphantly into the cremation flames wearing blue and purple glitter nail polish.

Knowing that Ken got what he wanted brings me a wave of peace. I learn that I can still serve as an advocate for someone who needs one, just like I did at Legal Aid. What I help Ken with might seem small to others, but to me, it is huge. I'm able to help him feel like an authentic version of himself. This is something I missed myself for so long, and now I can help other people do that when it matters most—when they have no more time to course correct or leave a mark on their own terms.

Death doulas get to honor the totality of the lived human experience for those of all identities, not just the ones we relate to or can understand. Individuals from communities that are marginalized especially deserve an advocate at the end of life. There are times where it is simply not possible to give the dying what they want, like the chance to assert their identity to an estranged family member. But focusing on the spirit of the request rather than the letter of it helps. When a particular type of flower is not available for a funeral, we adjust and pick something in the same family or color scheme. But when we are talking about bodies being misgendered or deadnamed at death, I will go to war for a client's wishes, to the extent they want me to. It is their death.

Too often parts of a person get erased in death because the biological family does not condone or support them, or because they were kept secret. All parts of our identity die along with us. We bury the whole person. If in death we could honor everyone for exactly who they were in life, we could work at breaking down the barriers that keep us separate from one another and separate from our complex humanity. And if in life we could live out loud the identities we carry and the expressions that scream from us, we could also shine light and love on the parts that others choose to hate. Fuck them. Do you, boo.

Chapter 11

Glimmer of Freedom

About eight months before the bottom fell out of my life, I arrived at work one Tuesday after a long weekend trip to the Mojave Desert. Honestly, I don't remember the trip that well. What I remember is the spike of dread as I sat down to the blinking red voicemail button on my office phone. As soon as I heard my old friend Silvia's voice asking me to call her, I could feel my pulse in my ears. Silvia was executive director at Legal Aid by then, and she'd been weathering a brutal round of budget cuts. I'd watched in fear as my colleagues were moved like chess pieces and older attorneys chose retirement. I had the suspicion that it would soon be my turn. With my door closed, I quickly changed out of my bike riding gear into my mishmash of lawyer work gear, took several deep breaths to calm myself down, and called her back.

"Alua." Silvia's tone was already apologetic.

My stomach dropped. "No," I said immediately. "Please don't, Silvia." Because she was my friend, I felt comfortable talking to the big boss like a petulant child.

Silvia did what she had to do. "You know there have been a lot of budget cuts and our fundraising has slowed. I've tried really hard to find a way for you to stay in your role, 'cause I know it gives you some freedom, but I can't anymore. We can keep you, but you'll have to start working at the Self-Help Center in the Inglewood Courthouse. It will only be six months, but you have to work full-time. Afterward we'll see if you can come back to your current position."

In the space of one phone call, the last bits of a life I could tolerate crumbled. The way my student loans were set up, quitting with no prospect for work wasn't an option, but I strongly considered it at the moment. I stared at the gray-brown carpet, tears clouding my vision. The carpet looked like the quicksand it felt like I was falling into. *I could make six months work, though—right? Right?*

Silvia continued, trying to inject some sunshine into the conversation. "I know that this isn't what you want. I'm sorry. But who knows, this could be the best thing that has happened to you yet!"

She was right, but not in the way she intended it. Sometimes best things seem like worst things until we let life unfold to reveal what is actually best. I didn't know that then, though. I was already stuck and about to get even more stuck.

My new role was to supervise volunteer attorneys and law students. There would be no direct client contact, which was the only aspect of my job that still nourished me. The strict schedule and the lack of interaction would be difficult at best. At worst, this would be the death knell for my spirit. As soon as I hung up the phone with Silvia, I sobbed.

I'd been sobbing a lot more lately. I tend to express all of my strong emotions, even joy, through tears, but now I was crying for any ole reason. One day a few months earlier, I cried because my bike tire went flat on the way to work. I was determined to soldier through and pretend nothing was wrong with me, but it was getting harder. I couldn't help but notice how irritable I was all the time, how lonely I felt even surrounded by friends.

With an immigrant daughter/strong Black woman's aversion to therapy operating at full tilt, I nonetheless decided, reluctantly, to pursue some "professional help." I thought that maybe what I needed was to vent. To bitch, to get it out of my system.

Within three sessions, the therapist diagnosed me with dysthymia—a persistent mild depression. I waved it away. I was $100k in student-loan debt, making $30k a year while Black in America and butting up against the insidious infrastructure of oppression. Who *wouldn't* be depressed? I'd been in and out of love again recently, and chalked up her diagnosis to heartache and misunderstanding. Clearly she didn't get me, but I thought no one did. Regardless, I kept working with her while pretending my need was temporary, and that my diagnosis was situational.

Within three months, she'd upgraded my diagnosis to a major depressive episode.

I *still* didn't think she knew what she was talking about.

Running on sheer self-denial, I survived my six-month stint at the Self-Help Center, but barely. I faux affectionately named my office The Dungeon. Days spent in The Dungeon turned into nights on the couch, drinking Cabernet Sauvignon and chain-smoking hash spliffs alone. The combo switched my brain and emotions off, numbing me long enough to avoid thinking about my life.

Every morning I woke up crying just as my alarm went off. Cursing the tears and the insomnia that persisted despite the hashish, I'd roll out of bed, hungover, and drag myself into the shower. I didn't care about being clean, but didn't want to stink. I'm too vain to stink, even depressed. I couldn't control my mind, which told me I was an utter failure who didn't deserve to have joy, but at least I could control my bodily odor. The tears mixed with the shower water. Standing in front of the closet unsure how to dress myself, I'd run out of energy for trying to look the part.

Hell, I'd run out of energy for everything. Dirty dishes spilled out of the sink onto the countertops and bedroom floor. My nails were chipped and jagged. The fridge held bags of decaying vegetables, mirroring what was happening inside my spirit. I only threw them away because they mocked me and reminded me of my inadequacy. The windows had been closed for weeks on end, and the only light that came in was from the broken blinds I didn't tell my landlord about. I'd grab the simplest item of clothing I could find in a dark color from the piles on the floor, pull my locs back, grab an overripe banana from the counter, and leave for my job at The Dungeon. No music in the car, just my sobs and the sounds of traffic. So many other people were going to work in the cars around me. Somehow they managed to get ready, drive, go to the office, feed themselves, and not hate their life—right? So why was I incapable of this simple act of being human?

Arriving around 8 A.M., I'd drive into a concrete parking structure, walk through metal detectors into the concrete building and straight to the basement, where I sat behind a desk in a tiny office. Then I'd put on a big smile. There were no windows to see the outside world. No sunshine. No nourishment. Every plant I brought there died. How could I thrive? I counted down the days till I could leave there, using the calendar as a carrot. Each day I survived brought me one day closer to leaving.

I withdrew from my friends, citing my new work schedule as the reason I was no longer available. In truth, I had no energy for anyone, and I didn't want them to see me like this. Broken. Sad. Despondent. And embarrassed. Simultaneously overwhelmed and numbed by people, sights, sounds. Conversation felt like rocket science. Even though I'd concentrate hard, I'd get confused about what people were saying halfway through, misread social cues, and stutter to respond appropriately. Nothing interesting to say, no joy to contribute. In my head, no one wanted to hang out with me anyway because I was the human equivalent of a wet dirty dish towel. I stayed indoors. Watching movies and TV has always bored me, so I'd stare into space, smoke more spliffs, and cry. I did not cry out of sadness. I cried out of desperation and despair.

Up until then, my life looked pretty great—at least from the outside. Meaningful work, flexible schedule, international travel, nice clothes, decent health, a great social life, fun boyfriends. I had a creative outlet in photography and a physical one in bike riding. My affordable apartment on the top floor of a duplex guesthouse in the middle of Los Angeles was shaded by orange and magnolia trees. It felt like a treehouse. My friends were eclectic, witty, rowdy, gorgeous. Yet something enormous was missing. I couldn't pinpoint it.

At thirty-four years old, I was still waiting for my life to begin, denying the fact that I was presently living it. The realization that *this* was my life shocked and saddened me. How did I become this? A shell of a human waiting for some distant day in the future when I could enjoy life. I'd always thought of myself as joyful, connected, vibrant, and engaged. I wanted a life I salivated over. One that dripped with love and magic, where I could live in rapture over the beauty of a caterpillar making its way down a vine. My life was the opposite of that. I wasn't sure why I was alive. What was the point?

I had *thought* that a life of service was the point. My parents had committed their lives to the service of Jesus Christ, uprooting their young children repeatedly to go where they were called to spread the gospel. Service was one of the core values they imparted to my sisters and me, simply by their example. By choosing to work in Legal Aid, I'd imagined myself carrying that vision forward. If I'd known that tying my life meaning to service would still have me end up crying all day, every damn day, I would at least have chosen also not to be broke. It all felt so empty. *I* was so empty.

For the last week of my tenure at The Dungeon, I cashed in my vacation time and the little bit of energy I had to go to the Burning Man festival. I'd never been, and I desperately needed it. I'd been an antisocial wreck for months, but the friends who hadn't given up on me packed up four vehicles of camping equipment, shade structures, tents, rebar, water, food, and our favorite outrageous clothes.

Burning Man is an annual nine-day experimental city in the middle of a dried-out lake bed in Nevada, built from scratch each year, including massive art installations, roads, street signs, homes, roller-skating rinks, a post office, medics, and a facsimile police force. It's also torn down after every festival. It's an inspiring celebration of humanhood, artistic expression, community, and pure freedom. Suffice it to say that in a desert, where nothing grows, it is a microcosmic playground where you will find exactly what you are looking for, but perhaps not the way you imagined.

In 2012, the first year of seven I attended, over 75,000 people descended upon Black Rock Desert with the shared principles of radical inclusion, radical self-reliance, radical expression, leaving no trace, and immediacy. There is an inherent magic in joining with people who are also committed to their personal freedom and the ecstasy of community. Having forgotten the methylsulfonylmethane (MSM) nutritional supplement I take daily, I overheard on our first night our camp neighbors talking about the extras they had brought. They shared it with me. Forgetting my hang-ups about my body weight that I still had despite my rapidly thinning frame, I let a petite man named Twilight lift my body over his with his legs alone in free-form acro yoga, twisting my body into shapes I hadn't previously thought possible. Each night the city lit up with thousands of bold, bright colored lights on bicycles, art cars, and humans in ethereal costumes worn for pure pleasure. Headdresses, bejeweled boots, coats decorated with illumination for the cold nights. I danced daily till dawn, laughed in the temple reserved for grief, cried in hammocks, and partied like it was 1999 even though it was 2012.

There were so many cures for restlessness at Burning Man that I needed to prioritize rest. Otherwise, I'd say yes to every offer in front of me, going on adventures that lasted all day and night. After all, part of the beauty of Burning Man lies in its impermanence. If you wanted to see that big piece of art, you had to go. They started burning the bigger structures on Friday, and by the end, there would be nothing left. Get out, go see, go play. Grab your joy right in front of you, because soon it will be gone forever.

One night around three, having a smoke by my bike outside of a raging party, I met and fell in infatuation with a Black bike messenger named Pascha. We roamed the playa till the sun came up. The next day, he returned for more adventures and we separated for dinner and to put on some clothes—all day he'd been naked except for a tool belt. Later, he was to come find me, but a dust storm brewed, blocking vision and masking everything more than an arm's length away. He never showed up. I was devastated.

Nonetheless, for the first time in years, I felt alive. My curiosity spark, which had grown dangerously dim, flared bright. Everywhere you looked there were things to be curious about: How did they make this massive beautiful structure? What in west Hades is that person wearing? Could I climb that big piece of art? What did the camp name Porn & Donuts mean? (Turns out, they served hot donuts and showed vintage silent porn between midnight and 2 A.M. I love donuts, so I stayed for a show.)

But most of all: Who *were* these people? So seemingly comfortable in their skin, in this life? And where were they in the default world? I suspected many came here because it was one of the only places they felt comfortable enough to be exactly who they were. They didn't come to let their freak flag fly, because none of us were freaks here. We were normal. And there was nothing wrong with any of us—we just lived in a society that didn't match our ideals.

At Burning Man, I was beginning to understand the question I'd been asking myself—what is wrong with me?—was incorrect. The problem wasn't me. The problem was society. It was okay if I couldn't live a life that was based on society's ideals. They weren't mine. Like the glorious structures I had just watched smoke and smolder to the ground, only to be reborn next year, I could start all over.

On our sixteen-hour drive back to Los Angeles after the Burn, I turned on my phone for the first time in a week. A voicemail notification flashed: the human resources department at Legal Aid.

I was needed at The Dungeon for an additional three to six months.

Time stopped. My mouth went dry. Fight-or-flight hormones raged. I felt like an anvil had landed on my chest. Freeze. Then, a voice inside. *No,* I said to myself. There was no way I could agree. In fact, there was no way I could go back at all.

Without a second thought, I muttered aloud to my sleepy and dreamy friends in the car, "I'm never stepping foot in that place again. I'll die if I do."

I meant it. Now that I had a glimpse of what life could be, I couldn't go back. I didn't yet know my way through but had to trust that life would hold me. There was no other choice. My life depended on not returning to Legal Aid as a lawyer.

Dora is in her late sixties and bald when we meet. Sixth-generation Mexican American and heavyset with thick, tortoise-shell glasses, she is confined to her bed in a luxury high-rise building in Los Angeles, incurably ill with bladder cancer. Her bedroom walls are decorated with expensive art in sleek, black frames: a minimalist's dream just like the rest of her home, full of clean lines, contrasting colors, mirrors, and a whole lot of glass. It is the sort of house that says, "I do not have to deal with small children."

Dora's end of life plans are complete. She's shared financial information with her grown kids, as well as the location and contents of her will. She's declined curative treatment, and her children know to prioritize quality of life, not quantity, in making decisions about her care. She's been clear she wants to die at home, as peacefully as bladder cancer will allow. Her body disposition plans are set, as well as the outfit she will wear at her funeral. She's checked off nearly all the items on her end of life planning list, so I wonder what is still undone in her life and why she has called me here. When I put this question to Dora, she asks me for support in "whatever else I might be overlooking as I prepare to die."

I sit on the Lucite chair closest to her bed, which faces a majestic balcony. The first female advertising executive at a mid-level agency, she has spent the majority of her life killing it at the office rather than being with her children—latchkey kids of the 1980s. She seems conflicted as she tells me all of this, repeatedly falling back on terms like *wasting* and *spending* to describe her time. They are evidence of the worldview she's about to leave behind.

I've noticed that the English language uses the verbs *spend, waste,* and *save* when talking about two things: time and money. But time is the only real currency we've got. The true cost of anything is how much life we give in exchange for it. We exchange time for money when we go to work. We exchange it for love when we release oxytocin with people who make us emit it. We exchange time for accomplishment when we finish a puzzle that's been sitting in the closet. It's a finite resource, but with no telling how much of it we've got. For Dora, now at the end of her life, she wonders if she exchanged time for the wrong thing.

"I never wanted to have children," Dora reveals to me with a sigh. "And I've never actually admitted that to anyone." We are alone. I am looking through Dora's advance planning document to see if anything needs some clarification.

This revelation comes out of left field, and I am careful to monitor my facial expression. I am not surprised that she didn't want kids, but I am surprised that she admitted it. Of the remaining taboos, admitting you didn't want to have your kids remains potent.

"Obviously I love them and I am glad they are here, but I did it because I thought I was supposed to. There wasn't much of a choice." Dora pauses. "I'm sorry, I shouldn't have said that."

She doesn't look sorry. In fact, she looks noticeably lighter.

"It's okay," I assure her. "If it's on your heart, I'd rather you say this now than not at all. And I'm really grateful that you feel comfortable enough to share this with me. I can imagine it's hard to say." I am not going to judge her choices as a human, and I also believe a lot more people who have children feel this way and never say.

We talk for a few more hours. Dora shares that she'd intended to stay at home to raise her children once she'd had them. After all, she was born in the late 1940s, and that's what most women of her generation did. But an absentee alcoholic ex-husband had made that impossible. Dora wanted her kids to have opportunities to grow into loving, successful contributors to society. She wanted to give them the chance to be their own people. So she leaned into the type of woman she became enamored with growing up: the kind who wore pants and went to an office every day. Women were newly allowed in executive workspaces back then. The idea of it was exciting to Dora.

Turns out, she was a marvel at it.

Dora wasn't present for much of the younger years of her children's lives, content as she was with her job and with being an early model for high-achieving, single working mothers—which was virtually nonexistent at the time. She raised her kids in a nice neighborhood in a spacious home with endless after-school activities, private lessons, the works, which was possible only because of her high-paying job. Dora's proud of this. Looking at her home and her neat, detailed death plan, I get a sense of what she brought to her career, as well as what her career has given her. Still, she seems unwilling, or even unable, to take uncomplicated pride in it and expresses guilt over not spending more of her time with the children.

Dora and I chat about the societal expectation of women and people with uteruses to have children. There is an inherent distrust and suspicion of those of us who don't have children or those who don't center them. Are we broken? Selfish? Greedy? Serial killers? For people with uteruses, it's expected that we want to use them to create more life. But what if the purpose of the life of a person with a uterus is not solely to use it to give birth? Perhaps I am content to bleed monthly for forty-plus years because it fascinates me and I can marvel at the design of my body, which marks the cycles of the moon through blood.

Cautiously, I ask Dora why she had children and what they'd

brought her. Even with the permission to speak candidly, it's still a delicate conversation. Whenever someone asks me, as a child-free woman, why I haven't yet had kids, I turn the question back on them, recognizing that my decision places me in the category of a woman who doesn't hold as much value as those who have birthed to some people. A woman I know once jokingly suggested that I ride my bike through a busy intersection before her, because I had no children. I didn't find it funny.

"I don't know," Dora responds. "We have great relationships, though, so I don't know what I'm getting on about." She starts to dismiss the conversation, but I lean in physically, listening with my whole body, and that cues her to continue. "But they weren't everything to me. They weren't enough. I feel terrible saying that, but they weren't. I feel bad I wasn't there for them more growing up, but I only feel bad because I didn't want to be there. They turned out fine. With or without me." She looks out the window while she talks. "They weren't the center of my life," she confesses. "I've listened to my friends talk almost exclusively about their children for decades. I chime in because I think I sound like a monster if I don't."

Dora is seeking greater understanding of her time on Earth. She had interests that went unexplored, curiosities that went unfilled, potential that went untapped. She explains that aside from her job, she'd put much of what she'd wanted aside for her children. She regrets that now at the end of her life.

As we talk, I notice something happening to Dora. She is sitting up straighter, and even though she is weak from her illness, she is growing more and more animated. I can almost see the weight of each societal expectation leaving her tired frame, one by one. In her heart, she is not ashamed of how she chose to spend her time. She has been made to feel that way by a society that did not share her priorities. I am glad Dora is unburdening herself before her death. It's more proof that people get a lot more honest when they know there is nothing left to lose.

My work with Dora presented an added dimension to the death work doulas often do. Sometimes the paperwork, plans, and documents are already firmly in place and there are no glaring omissions. Sometimes the client needs something else that's less tangible and hard for them to describe, though the yearning for it is there. Dora may not have known exactly what the "whatever else" was she was looking for when she hired me, but she sensed she was overlooking . . . something. In the end, she wanted clarity on the purpose of her life.

Yet if Dora had told me that at the start, I would have balked at the suggestion that I could assist her. I don't have the hubris to believe I can help people uncover their purpose. For some, having a purpose has value. For others, the experience of being alive carries enough meaning. And at its root, it is an unanswerable question from the outside. Death can create the context for us to find meaning in our lives, but we must do the work ourselves, centering our values, our curiosity, and our contentment.

Through our conversation, Dora becomes clear about the purpose of her life: to follow her own joy. She had made cool people and modeled to them what it looked like for a mom to pursue a life not defined by them, despite what society told her. She was never looking for her children to bring *her* something, and she didn't get much out of motherhood. She wanted them to be their own people. She loved them but they did not fill up or "complete" her—and that's okay. This realization brings Dora peace. And that's all that matters.

Dora died a few months into our work together. Her last months were spent on the little things that brought her pure gratification. With her taste buds mostly destroyed from years of chemotherapy, she relied heavily on her sense of smell to get pleasure from food. She ate. A lot. As much as she could stand, given that she was ill and dying. Mostly fast food, which she'd eschewed for years while dieting, but also passion fruit soufflé and key lime pie.

She mentored a female junior advertising executive who used to be an intern when Dora was still working, helping the young mother to reconcile home and career. Dora started reading about mushrooms and found awe in the network of fungi upon which our natural world survives and thrives.

And she spent time with her children, who doted upon the dying mother who worked hard for most of her life to give them opportunities. Dora died clear about the purpose of her one life.

So many of us reach the end of our lives wishing we knew the particular reason we ever existed: our why, our "hero project," as explained by Ernest Becker in his book *The Denial of Death*, or the "aha moment" from Oprah. "The two most important days in your life are the day you are born and the day you find out why," Mark Twain said once, and a million high school seniors have repeated it on their yearbook pages since. Yet how many of us are living with Twain's words far, far in the distance, simply waiting for purpose to slap us across the face?

This is how I used to be. I searched so hard for my purpose that I practically thought it'd be gift-wrapped for me in a pretty box. I was convinced it was out there for me to find, like in a scavenger hunt. I conflated purpose with my job (hello, capitalism), I looked for it in Kip, and I knew I didn't want it to come out of my vagina. In time, I've come to believe my life does not have a *singular* purpose. Maybe yours doesn't either. The search for purpose itself—the worship of some glamorized future where everything suddenly makes sense—can be blinding. In my case, I was so busy looking for my purpose that I couldn't see it.

Yes, now that I'm a death doula, I have work that brings a fullness to my life beyond anything I could have imagined. I am grateful for it every day. But not nearly as grateful as I am for the mere opportunity to be briefly, perfectly human. To feel cold and grief, to experience awe and taste sugar on my tongue, to watch as light glints from a disco ball in the sun. This is important. Because while we are obsessed with trying to make meaning and purpose out of life, we can miss the experience of being here. We've got to find a good enough reason to give context to a life that can withstand waking up, working, eating, and pooping for roughly eighty-something years. If it brings you joy, make meaning out of the mundane. It's important to follow your curiosities and bliss wherever you can find it. It could be anywhere.

What if one of your purposes in life is to delight in the delicious syrup made with lavender and blackberries from your garden? Or to learn how to make macramé art finally? What if your joy in life is when Sisqó belts out the key change in "Thong Song" or you hear Juvenile call out *Cash Money Records taking over for the '99 and the 2000* just before the beat drops? What if what brings you purpose is reveling in the mysteries of life and the simplicities and perfection of nature? Would these be sufficient?

Most of us know what tickles us. We can identify activities, or parts thereof, which bring us wonder and bring us a feeling of flow and ease. And as we stumble upon new things, we know the undeniable instinct which says *lean into this*—to a person, an idea, a place, or a way we feel about ourselves. Yet so many of us wait to take that step toward it, procrastinating our whole lives long. We wait until tomorrow, but no one is ever guaranteed a tomorrow. The consequences for waiting can be irreversible.

Chapter 12

Stepping off the Wheel

At Burning Man, I'd remembered what tickled me, what it felt like to be present in my life. And I was no longer interested in waiting around for it. I called my therapist on the phone in an SOS emergency session and tearfully explained that I'd been asked to go back to The Dungeon.

"I can't go back. I'll die. I can't. I'll die," I sobbed and repeated. I lay prostrate on the cool bathroom floor, rubbing my finger into the grout until the skin was raw. I knew the words I ~~were~~ *was* speaking were truth.

Within a day, I was on a ninety-day medical leave of absence from work for clinical depression.

I clung to the opportunity with immense relief, mingled with shame. There is a luxury in stepping off the hamster wheel of work, but it comes with a heavy professional stigma. Lawyers don't take breaks. They certainly don't take them for mental health reasons. I still don't know a single lawyer who has taken a leave of absence or left the profession for their mental health—even though many of the lawyers I knew needed it.

At the time, I thought ninety days was excessive; I just needed a break to clear my head, regain perspective. But I would have rather been labeled depressed than dead. That's the ruthless binary of depression. It told me I had two options: "depressed" or "dead." There was no room for "hope." Depression suffocates it.

Office gossip had me pregnant, lying, or on leave to take care of a family member, and colleagues who became friends from Legal Aid called, trying to understand. It seemed no one could believe that my mental health had deteriorated to the point of disability. Honestly, neither could I. There was no way they could know. I'd gotten so good at masking my illness with smiles and deflecting attention that even my own family and friends were unable to help me.

My depression had become my little secret—one that I didn't keep well from those who knew me best. My family members were trying to get in, and I was keeping them out. I worried my parents would think they'd done something wrong or hadn't been enough for me. There were a lot of us kids, not a lot of money or time. I never wanted to be a bother. Perhaps this was middle-child syndrome, a title I share with Ahoba, the third of the four of us—some version of "I'm fine, don't worry about me. I don't have needs, I don't have desires. Don't forget about me, but don't fuss over me either."

Whenever my mother asked me how I was doing, I would say I was okay. "Just okay?" she'd respond. She knew something was wrong. I could hear the pleading in her voice for me to share more, but I also heard her natural mother's desire for me to be good or—even better—great. I'd rush her off the phone to avoid crying, because I knew her heart was breaking. My dad wanted us to be successful. My mom just wanted us to be happy. I was hurting them both.

It was only my fault, I reasoned. I had "done it to myself." My parents had given my sisters and me everything—not only life, but a *good* life. Safety, love, acknowledgment, private dates with my mom when we got our periods, road trips to Disneyland driven by my dad. They worked hard to make sure we had what we needed, even if that meant our new clothes came from Goodwill. Why, then, was it not enough? Did women my age living in Ghana have the luxury to be bored or depressed?

As it does in big families, gossip travels. I knew I was being talked about because one sister would have information that I'd only told another one. My sisters' voices were heavy with concern when we'd talk, and they'd steer the conversation back to me when I tried to deflect. Aba was the only one who lived near me. I think they agreed she'd be the emissary. She would say she was on the way to check on me and I'd tell her I wasn't home, knowing damn well I hadn't left the couch in days. I'd go as far as to park my car around the block in the event she dropped by. Once I watched her look over the gate while I peeked out of the broken window blinds. I was too proud to admit that I was hurting and ashamed that they knew anyway. But no one knew how bad it had gotten. I withdrew altogether, keeping them abreast of only my plans and safe arrivals, and very little else.

I certainly didn't tell them about Pascha. Within a few days I found the naked man I'd become infatuated with at Burning Man and lost in a dust storm. He'd placed a craigslist missed connection ad for me and a friend of mine had seen it: *Hi, your name begins with an A, you're from Ghana. I'm from Kentucky and my name begins with a P. I need you in my life, I hope you find this message and contact me. I tried to find your camp, but I have a feeling that you left during the white out. I loved your presence and want you so much, ciao for now.* Ah—a good old-fashioned distraction. And right around the time I was scheduled to do some highly inconvenient self-examination! I leapt at the chance.

Within two weeks of being granted a leave of absence, I was off to Portland on a one-way ticket to see Pascha for his birthday. He bought the ticket; I was his birthday gift to himself. Depression can happen anywhere, I decided, so I'd go be depressed in Portland instead. At least Pascha and I would have an opportunity to get to know each other. As usual, I hoped that I would be cured by his love, hoped he would save me from myself. I'd hoped for a full Disney ending—except with full frontal nudity.

In the real world, our romance lasted four days. I came off the pink infatuation cloud and crashed to Earth within minutes of our re-union, as we walked through the grocery store shopping for my stay. It finally hit me that I did not know this man I was staying with in a strange city. Black olives? Childhood trauma? Creamy or crunchy peanut butter? Arrest record? We filled our conversation with trivial-ities to cover up the fact that all I really knew about him was how his naked body looked covered in Burning Man's playa dust. We'd never had sex. Still, I'd willingly hopped on a one-way flight to a strange man in a strange land. Lust is a hell of a drug.

It wasn't Pascha's fault. A Black country boy from the sticks in Ken-tucky, he had lived all over Europe as a bike messenger and had a bike messenger body—lean, muscular, stacked. He spoke fluent Russian, German, Flemish, and Spanish, all in a country drawl, and studied Russian in college. And he played the cello. I was as good as done.

But he was twenty-four years old—I'd often dated younger men, but this was young even by my standards. And as a man who moved often and didn't stay anywhere long enough to make friends, his am-bivalence about my staying with him hurt. A lot. He barely talked to me while I was there, overwhelmed by my presence, but would beg for me to stay when I suggested that I should leave. I was over the hot-cold game that he seemed to be playing. I like to know that a man likes me. He preferred to hunt mushrooms in the woods alone than talk to humans. His apartment was the size of a shoebox, which would have only fit my jewelry and his cello. Hell, I brought more things to Portland on this trip than he'd likely owned in his lifetime. I couldn't settle into his life. I wasn't settled in mine.

Four days after I arrived, I moved into a hotel nearby and cried for a few more days, hoping the tears were just garden-variety sexual frustration. (We *still* hadn't had sex—there was no heart alignment.) Pascha was supposed to be another distraction, but the distractions weren't working anymore. My depression was deepening. And for the first time, I couldn't drink it away, travel it away, shop it away, fuck it away.

Thinking I'd be in Portland for a while, I'd sublet my apartment in Los Angeles. That meant I was free to go wherever I wanted until my medical leave of absence was over. But where to? I'd packed enough so that I could flex my limited wardrobe—a pair of expensive Camper shoes from Mallorca, and one fancy dress in case an event arose that allowed me to put my pretty on. After years of traveling with just a backpack, I understood minimalism, but I didn't like it. I'd also packed three books, a journal, and a large rose quartz crystal, which I clung to when it felt like I was slipping into darkness again. It came everywhere with me.

Not knowing where to go next, I sought out an energy healer who told me that I should not go back home. "Keep going," she said during a Reiki session. But I was at the end of my road. I didn't know who I was or what I wanted. I couldn't feel anything; depression had dulled my senses. I couldn't feel myself.

Walking back to the hotel after my session, the rain started. Soft at first, then it quickly grew to a thunderous downpour. I hadn't packed a raincoat and had nothing to hold over my head. I was not far, or so I thought, so I walked swiftly in the rain but the sidewalk ran out. Gingerly, I walked along the side of the freeway hoping a car wouldn't splash or hit me and that the hotel would soon appear like the Emerald City in *The Wizard of Oz*. Sade's *Soldier of Love* album had just dropped, so I marched the streets in the rain listening to the album, with the title song on repeat: *I've lost the use of my heart. But I'm still alive.*

I'd bet on love and lost. I'd bet on a career and lost. I'd bet on joy and lost. I'd bet on a dry fucking afternoon and I was drenched, lost on foot along the freeway in Portland with nowhere to go. Even the skies had opened up to let the clouds grieve alongside me. Desperate once again, rain and tears mixed, dripping down my chin, Sade in my ear reminding me that I was a soldier. She'd never lied to me before but this was a stretch. I was a failure.

After a few wrong turns, the path to the hotel became clear again.

Once inside I dried myself, warmed up, took two shots of whiskey, and thought about my options. My mom had been begging me to go visit her, but I didn't want her to see me like this. I was convinced it would kill her. Same with my sisters.

This was my self-denial talking. My family, then as now, just wants what's best for me. But my inner drive to make them proud made me turn my face away from them. I was supposed to achieve, to fulfill the immigrant parents' dream of their children reaching a higher social class, to excel in everything I touched. They were *so proud* that I was a lawyer. When I graduated law school, they threw me a party, inviting the other Ghanaians in Colorado to share in our success. After all, they *all* had a lawyer now, not just my parents. My accomplishment was for the community. How could I look all of them in the face and tell them the truth? That I hated being a lawyer, and that a lawyer's life was slowly killing me.

Instead, I paced and returned a call from my friend Kristin, who was curious about how my romance was going. I did not admit that I had just been lost, wet, and sobbing, but did indicate that I was free to travel. I tried to make it seem like I was charmingly on the road, and not hungry for direction. She invited me to her home in Colorado. I eagerly accepted. Another adventure; another distraction. I would deal with myself at some point. Just not today. I wasn't ready.

Depression is a liar. It tells you that there is no hope. That tomorrow will be exactly the same. That you are a burden. That it is contagious. That no one cares, that it is your fault. That since you weren't strong enough to stave it off, you're not strong enough to get well again, and that you don't know what "well" is. That you don't deserve it.

But most of all, depression tells you that no one can understand and that no one can help. Not even—or especially—those closest to you, who love you most.

When Martha calls me, she is not ready to speak. I answer the

phone while cleaning my apartment on a Tuesday afternoon, drop-
ping my mop when I hear the cries on the other end. I sit on the
floor. I wasn't expecting this type of call, but death doulas are generally ready to handle difficult emotions with zero notice. Between
strangling sobs, she tells me that her son Sean has just been found by
his roommate, dead on the floor of his bedroom from an apparently
self-inflicted gunshot wound to the head.

He was thirty-one years old.

Understandably, Martha can't make sense of what she's heard or
what this reality means. Sean was her only child. He'd moved to
Utah a couple of years prior to get closer to outdoor sports and a
slower pace of life than in Los Angeles.

"I'm sorry. I thought I was doing better," she says, each phrase
punctuated by a gulp. It sounds as though she is trying to swallow
marbles. It has only been a few hours since Sean's roommate has
called. Her son's body might even still be in the apartment, waiting for removal by the coroner's office. I remind Martha that Sean's
death is still so fresh and she hasn't had any time to assimilate the
information yet: her son is dead, and he'd likely died by his own
hand. How is anyone ever supposed to get their head around that
news, even decades after the fact, let alone hours? It's a wonder she
isn't comatose, sitting and staring at nothing. Instead, she has called
for support.

Some people are leveled by news of death, others spring into action. Neither is better than the other. Martha is clearly the latter,
though. As soon as she heard from Sean's roommate, she immediately contacted Sean's father, from whom she had been divorced
for decades, as well as her siblings. One of them suggested she seek
support and Martha did a Google search to find me. I am her fifth
phone call.

A death doula probably isn't someone most think of after a sudden death, given that most of our work is done with people with
awareness of their approaching death. Since we work with the dying

person and their community, our services are helpful to all impacted by a death, even when it is sudden. At the very least, we can be a nonjudgmental support person along the journey. A few joint deep breaths later, Martha is ready to move into action.

"Okay, so what do I need to do now?" she asks.

"Do you need a day or two to be with this news before you try to do anything?" I suggest.

"No. I don't."

I hear her loud and clear. I can appreciate a woman who knows herself, despite what I think is best. I ask if she wants to go to Utah or if she wants to stay in L.A. Understandably, Martha wants to go be with her son, identify his body, and be among his things. Her voice cracks when she talks about seeing his art. And she talks fast and angrily about the gun she didn't know he owned.

I ask how she wants to proceed. The type of work we do together after this phone call depends on how much Martha wants to do herself, since the work of wrapping up affairs could be done with minimal involvement on her part. I could also advise her over the phone, creating a schedule for consultations to answer her questions, or put her in touch with a graduate of the Going with Grace doula training program who is in Utah through a doula matching service to put boots on the ground.

"I need to do it all. I can't just sit here. I just need someone to tell me what to do and to lean on while I do it. Is that okay? Can you do that? Can you hold me up?" Her voice has grown thin, tight, and high, pleading.

"I'll do my best." *Strong back, soft front*: this is the doula motto taught to me by my teacher Olivia.

I hang up the phone after setting up a schedule for phone consultations over the next month. I want to wait a few days to allow Martha to think about our arrangement, but she assures me that she'll feel the same in a couple of days. We can make hasty decisions after a death and I want Martha to be as clear-headed as possible before signing a contract. I try to remind my clients of this, as they often make fast and expensive decisions with funeral homes shortly after a death. There is no rush. Let the death simmer a bit. The services will be there, and grief will still be there.

In the weeks after Sean's death, Martha rents a monthlong sublet in Salt Lake City half a mile from his apartment, finds a funeral home to reconstruct his face so she can see his body, and arranges his funeral. She contacts the police department to make sure that they keep and destroy the gun Sean used to end his life. Before she arrives, she finds a carpet service to rip it all out so she doesn't have to see any blood-stains on the floor. She also boxes up his clothes and books, forwards his mail, sells his climbing gear and mountain bike, and frames his drawings to keep. Sean's roommate helps by telling her which of Sean's remaining belongings he wants. She donates the rest. Grief energizes some. It annihilates many others. As far as checking things off the "wrapping-up affairs" checklist, Martha is cruising. Emotionally, however, she is in choppy waters.

"I can't stop wondering if I could have stopped him. Is this normal?" she asks, unprompted, as we talk through closing out his social media accounts. Martha was able to log in using the password to his phone, which she found on his computer, which did not have a pass code. This is a small victory. Martha uncovers a string of direct messages with a woman alluding to a recent breakup. She didn't know Sean was seeing anyone. As expected, she's trying to make her brain compute how her son made a choice this drastic. There are no clues she can find, no answers to be had. All of the answers died along with Sean.

A slightly melancholy kid, Sean was well loved by friends until he got to middle school. There he'd been bullied mercilessly by his peers for his lanky build, acne, and love of dirt, rocks, and farm animals. Formerly an engaged student, his grades tanked. He stopped talking to Martha, spending whole weekends asleep and mumbling to communicate his desires. He wouldn't eat anything she prepared and he'd started drinking water directly from the faucet. She figured his body was either drowning in teenage hormones or he was depressed. In some cases, those are indistinguishable. She decided to wait it out.

As far as Martha knew, he'd "grown out of it." He'd gone to a few years of community college and discovered his love for anime and rock climbing. Unable to make a living as a visual artist, he'd taken restaurant kitchen jobs to pay the bills so he could continue drawing and climb when weather permitted. He'd recently lost his job. But he told his mom that everything was okay and from afar, all she had to rely on was his word. I felt a pang, reminding me of my mother's concerned voice over the phone, helplessly repeating "Just okay?" Even if Martha had been there, Sean likely would have been able to mask the gravity of his illness. It's a skill for those of us that struggle with mental health.

Over beers one night, Sean's roommate tells Martha that after Sean lost his job he spent most days on the couch playing the video games that were the inspiration for his art. He'd retreat to his bedroom at night, sleep till late afternoon, and start playing games again till the wee hours of the morning. He'd stopped hanging out with his rock-climbing buddies and dishes piled up in his room. His roommate was starting to tire of the lack of cleanliness, but gave Sean some grace because it was clear he was "going through something."

"But how was I to know he'd kill himself?" she spits at me, exasperated.

"Exactly. You couldn't." How is anyone ever to know?

Given a particular set of circumstances, isolation, and lack of mental health support, I think quite a few people could be capable of this same thing. Including those who don't look like it. Including me. We all pretend that we are immune from that level of despair and hopelessness. We are not. We are all just one phone call, one diagnosis, one chemical imbalance, one bankruptcy, one accident away from a physical or mental disability that might make us not want to live anymore.

There isn't much I can tangibly offer Martha. Her rational mind knows that there is no way she could have stopped Sean, yet her mother's heart believes that she should have known her son was hurting. She also feels guilty that she is angry with Sean for choosing suicide. All I can do is listen, validate her struggles, offer resources, and bear witness to her pain and confusion.

In her more reflective moments, Martha shares her shame. The swallowing-marbles sound in her throat is back. She is ashamed that her son has died this way and worries about the stigma. "What tone should the funeral take?" "Should we acknowledge it?" "Everyone who will be there already knows." "Should we mention it in his obituary? Then the whole world will know."

Questions like these are impossible for me to answer *for* Martha. Her levels of acceptance around mental health differ from mine, so it's important that she honor her needs. I encourage her to center herself and Sean in her decision-making, as the funeral ritual is often just as much for the living as it is to honor the life of the person who has died. What would serve her best? And what would cause harm? Under what circumstances would she want people to know his cause of death? And why? Or why not?

It saddens me that a decision like suicide is one that we feel the need to hide in the dark. I remind Martha that Sean's death, even at his own hand, was still a death worthy of the grief, loss, and reverence we pay to other deaths. If he had a disease of the body that progressed untreated until it killed him, there would be no shame. We are quick to say that someone who died after a painful illness is "free of their suffering and pain," but we don't offer the same platitudes after a death by suicide, even though it is true. Sean had a disease of the mind, which in the throes of depression, rarely feels like a disease. It feels like the truth. A serious depression is what killed Sean. Most suicide is the result of an illness. We don't talk about it as such.

Not all parts of the work of a death doula are love and light. Death work encompasses the tough, gritty, terrorizing, and painful deaths. Babies die; there are bloody homicides, overdoses, preventable accidents, devastating circumstances. People die from all types of things, not just illness, where we have a chance to say goodbye and regard it as a natural process of the body. All command attention, grief, softness, and mercy. And all are sacred, deserving of honor and sanctity.

Until recently the common language used to classify a death by suicide was that the person "committed" suicide, because it was deemed a criminal act in many parts of the world, and still is in Ghana. It's obviously not punishable, because when it is successful, there is no one left to prosecute. Suicide is no longer considered a crime in the United States, at least in the legal sense—although some states still have "attempted suicide" laws on the books—but the stain remains. "Death by suicide" is a more accurate way to reflect that it is just another way people die. Much like death by cancer, death by drowning, death by angry bull. It is not a crime. It is a way out of a painful life.

Societally, we have internalized some of depression's lies—that sadness is wrong, that it is bad, that it is not valuable. That it needs to be made "better." We celebrate wellness and leave no space for sorrow, brokenness, grief, or anything other than "I'm fine" when the truth is that life is complicated, painful, and difficult. Whole humans feel a whole range of emotions, but we applaud only half of them, driving our negatively perceived emotions deep into hiding for fear of judgment. There, they are safe to fester and grow stronger, which in turn drives us to hide them more.

People say "you are not alone" all the time, but the loneliness of depression is cavernous, blanketing, deafening—so much louder than the voices from the outside. Paradoxically, we *all* feel alone at our lowest moments. And so we hide, we hide, we hide. We hide until we cannot bear the voices inside anymore. Until we become walking ghosts. Until we hit rock bottom. Until someone sees how bad we are hurting. Until we let them help. Or until we don't. And then we die.

Chapter 13

Troubled Legacies

The things we try to hide in life come out in death—unresolved conflicts, long-held regrets, dark secrets. No matter how far we run from these demons, they have a way of coming back to haunt us on our deathbed. If we die with unfinished business, it becomes the burden of loved ones left behind. Wounds created by the dying aren't erased by their death. Sometimes, they cut deeper. The urge to run away from our secrets only demonstrates the power they have over us.

What if we practiced saying the scary thing, owning the shitty thing, showing up to the challenging thing? It's daunting work to be done on the deathbed, so why not take our opportunities in life? A big part of embracing our mortality means reconciling our relationships. When looking at yourself on your deathbed in your mind's eye, who is around you? Who is choosing to be there? Who is choosing *not* to be there and why? It's important to acknowledge the difficult relationships we've had and the tricky emotions they bring. Acknowledging our resentment, anger, betrayal, and rejection to ourselves is a solid place to begin. And it's even more helpful if we can address it with the people who have caused or received it. Sometimes it's just too late. Nearing the end of life, I have observed that people are concerned with three major questions:

Who did I love?

How did I love?

Was I loved?

The answers are as varied as the individual lives themselves. But they point to the truth. From the minute we are recognized as humans—whether at conception, in the womb, or at birth—we begin leaving a legacy. We leave a legacy with every word, every smile, every action, and every inaction. It's not optional. Our legacies can be big or small. What matters is that we will all touch someone. How we do it is up to us.

When we die, that legacy will be revealed. The results are not always positive.

A few years ago, I read an obituary that took my breath away. The surviving children of a woman who died absolutely obliterated their mother, for the whole world to read. She had been torturous to them their entire childhoods and continued her abuse of them as adults, exposing everyone she met to her evil, violence, criminal activity, vulgarity, and "hatred of the gentle or kind human spirit." They wrote, in part, "we celebrate her death from this earth and hope she lives in the afterlife reliving each gesture of violence, cruelty, and shame that she delivered on her children." I had never read anything so scathing or rooted in deep agony.

The obituary appeared in print and online only briefly before it was removed. I will never know why it was taken down, but I wonder if having it out there, even momentarily, gave some modicum of closure and peace to the woman's children, signaling their nightmare was over. Perhaps it could also have been taken down because of the caustic nature of their feelings, which highlight a societal taboo: we are not to speak ill of the dead. When we can't say something nice, we are taught to say nothing at all. This suppresses the very human need to grieve difficult relationships.

While I've certainly seen a few in my work as a death doula, it's rare that people welcome death knowing that they've wronged others without attempting to make some type of amends. Unfortunately, sometimes it's just too late.

I've also sat with clients who tearfully confessed to me that they didn't know what to do with their feelings about an estranged family member who was dying, even if there was an attempt at reconciliation. They wanted to know: How do we mourn when someone with a troubled legacy leaves this earth?

When Janet first calls me, she is lighthearted, professional, and straight to the point. It is clear that she wants to handle some business, and I'm surprised when I learn the heaviness of it. After his referral to hospice, her dying father, James, revealed to her that he has five additional children that she never knew about. As the only child of her mother and father, who were married, Janet, forty-two, is frustrated, hurt, and angry. And now James wants her to work with her newly revealed siblings to coordinate his needs at the end of his life.

My reaction can be summed up in one word: *Eek!* I've never been called to support such dense family dynamics, and this feels *way* outside the scope of my work, more a job for a mediator or family therapist than a death doula. There are always family disputes at the end of life, but until this moment, I've never dealt with newly discovered siblings, secret mistresses, hidden families.

The siblings are all aware that his life will soon be ending. James wants peace, Janet tells me—both within himself for the secrets he's kept during his life, and also among his children. Ironically, his need for peace has caused turmoil in Janet. She'd assumed that she would be the one to make his end of life decisions, manage his finances, and plan his burial and services. But now she has to coordinate with five strangers toward whom she already holds animosity—through no fault of theirs. Janet is also grateful that she hasn't had to discuss any of this with her mother, who died nine years prior. She's angry with her father, who has tried to explain his decision, but—understandably—nothing he says is good enough.

"I don't know how I'm going to do this, Alua. He's dying and now I have to clean up his fucking mess." Elsewhere in our conversation, Janet has been cool and collected about the situation she's found herself in, but the facade has dropped.

I have no idea what to say. *Acknowledge and validate*, I remind myself. I try to imagine what it would feel like to be a daughter learning this about her father, and find that I cannot do it. Rather than rely on empathy, I choose compassion. "That's completely understandable," I manage. "This is a tough situation."

"I need to talk to them but don't know how," Janet continues. "I don't want anything to do with them, and at this moment I don't want anything to do with *him*. But I don't have a choice. I'm not going to abandon him on his deathbed. How are we going to do this?" Even in her anger and frustration, she is still using *we* to include everyone, and I think she also means me.

In this situation, I am in over my head. I offer to help her find a mediator or a family therapist, but Janet insists she wants to work with me. So I offer the skills I have. "Would it help if I explained the duties which arise at the end of life to all of you together and help you decide which ones you'd like to take on?"

"Yes." She pauses. "I think."

We arrange a sibling video meeting online where they will listen to the different duties necessary to wrap up a life and figure out who will take on which responsibility. Foolishly, I allot only an hour on a Saturday afternoon for this work of a lifetime.

Our intention for the meeting is education and collaboration, and we start with introductions. Some of the siblings know of each other, and a few have met, but none are friendly. My quick math determines that some were born when others were in utero or very young. They range in age from almost fifty to their thirties. All were born during James's marriage to Janet's mother. It is, in every sense of the word, a clusterfuck.

Before everyone gets a chance to talk, tensions are running high. There is a lot of huffing, puffing, and eye rolling. The Grief Olympics have commenced. The Grief Olympics result when someone insists that they are hurting more than someone else because of the circumstances of a death. They often begin with "at least you . . ."

> At least you didn't have him around for as long as I did.
> At least you had him for more than birthdays and some holidays.
> At least you knew who he was.
> At least you didn't have to learn he wasn't who you thought he was.
> At least you got to live with him.
> At least you didn't have to watch him get sick.
> At least you knew he was sick.

It is a resentment chorus, with each singing the refrain louder than the next. From my outsider's perspective, they are all entitled to their grief just as it is. Everyone is. There is no gold medalist in grief. To regroup, I call for a break to reset the energy. We are only twenty minutes into the meeting. It is going south fast.

I immediately call Janet and offer the number of a mediator I've used before in case she wants to scrap the whole thing. This feels voyeuristic and I'm out of my league, but I can't leave them like this. Their collective pain is more than I know how to handle, and I fear I am making the situation worse. Janet strongly disagrees and she wants me to stay in the conversation. She wants to hear how the others feel about her father's death. She wants to handle what her father hadn't during his life. She doesn't want to bear his death alone. And she thinks I can hold it all. Thirty jumping jacks later, we get back on the video call with a game plan.

As we begin, I ask each sibling to remember that the other is grieving, and that we have a common goal. Then I turn it over to Janet, who thanks them for their presence and admits that she's held a feeling of superiority since she is the only "legitimate" child. The Grief Olympics threaten to get started again when the oldest sibling chimes in with a claim to the longest relationship with their father, but Janet disarms it with an apology—a whole hero. Tensions subside. They listen to Janet's sadness over the impending death, but also her relief at finally having people to shoulder the responsibility of her father with her. Only children bear a particular weight when their parents die. Slowly they each share their grief at not having relationships with each other and their frustrations with their father for not introducing them earlier. They've found a common ground. An hour and twenty minutes into the meeting, we finally have an opening to discuss what we've gathered for.

They are all clear that they want to honor James's decision to die at home. Since Janet has had extensive conversations with him about his medical treatment and lives in the same city, it is agreed that she will be assigned his medical power of attorney. She will move in and provide care, receiving respite from a sibling who lives in the neighboring town. When talk of his financial power of attorney comes up, everyone bristles, until it is agreed that the accountant sibling should be listed on the forms, while all the financial decisions will be made in concert. I don't offer to facilitate those calls because I value my peace of mind.

Two and a half hours in, we are finally making progress, with many small duties left to divvy up.

Nearing the end of the call, one sibling asks whether their mother would be allowed to come to the service. She'd had a romantic relationship with James and wants to say goodbye. Janet seethes. She's barely begun to reconcile that she has siblings and doesn't want to also have to come face-to-face with these women who are not her mother. After a strained exchange, they agree that their mothers can come if they want, as long as everyone agrees to remain peaceful. This is particularly painful for Janet, as her mother is no longer alive. Yet it is also a relief that her mother won't have to suffer the sight of the physical representations of her husband's infidelity. It would have been grief on grief on grief.

Almost four hours and many snack and jumping jacks breaks later, the goodbye has all the softness of a Brillo pad, but at least we were done. I'm amazed that they all stayed on the call.

Each sibling now has their individual work of grief ahead, plus the roles we'd assigned during the call. They each also have to start reconciling the secrets their father kept over his life and their individual paths to forgiveness. Or not. The death of someone does not require that we forgive them if it doesn't serve us. As long as we are at peace with the choice we have made, that's all that matters.

Two weeks later, Janet calls to let me know that her father died surrounded by the love and laughter of four of his six children at his bedside. They didn't have a chance to get much of his paperwork done or handle all his affairs, but they did start forming relationships. She is surprised to see her father's walk mimicked by one of her siblings and agrees to mentor a nephew. Together, they got to accompany the man who gave them all life to his death.

When someone dies who has hurt us, it's hard or confusing to know how to hold both grief and anger, or sorrow and relief. Or to give yourself permission to feel those feelings in different measures. Not everyone is sad when someone dies. Some are relieved. Not every loss is a loss, and grief doesn't always look like sadness. We need to make room for other responses to death, not just sadness and despair, to honor the lushness of the human experience.

Legacies of pain and hurt don't always look the same. For example, my client Jack, eighty-eight, was a raging racist. He was also beloved by his family, who hired me.

Jack's sons, Andrew and John, call me with a disagreement about whether or not their father needs additional pain medication. Their wives have encouraged them to get my take.

Jack has been complaining about pain to his son John, who just wants him to be comfortable. Because he isn't presenting any signs of pain, however, Andrew's worried about potential opiate addiction. Both seem genuinely concerned about their father, and treat the other with respect, but neither will budge. In the background of the phone call, I can hear Jack moaning in frustration.

After making sure Andrew and John are clear that death doulas do not administer pain medication because it is medical treatment, and that I will defer to what the doctors suggest, they insist on hiring me. They want help understanding the next steps, and they want to get on the same page. I agree to come meet them. Andrew greets me warmly in a light blue, button-down shirt and khaki pants outside the chain-link fence of Jack's house with a sheepish look that immediately puts me on alert. "I really should have told you before you came," he says, "but my dad is kinda racist."

I look at him blankly and try to take in this huge fucking fact that he neglected to mention. He knows I'm Black. He could have saved me the hour and a half drive outside of Los Angeles and whatever emotional gymnastics I'll have to perform to get through this.

"*Kinda* racist?" I ask. "A little racist is a whole racist as far as I'm concerned. I didn't agree to this." I've got limited time on Earth and prefer to not spend *any* of it with people for whom my mere existence evokes hatred.

"I know. I'm sorry." He appears genuinely pained. "We didn't know what else to do and we didn't think anyone else could help us. Plus, you're just going to talk to *us*, right?"

I purse my lips, take a deep breath, and take stock. He's right that I am here to support the sons, and I've already driven the whole way. I am seething, but I agree to go inside *only* to talk to Andrew and John. Jack is sleeping in the living room, so Andrew suggests we go in through the back door, reminiscent of the help in a not-so-long-ago time in America.

"No way. This isn't 1929. I'm going in the front door." I'm curt and already regretting my decision to stay. Squirming, Andrew quickly recognizes his mistake and apologizes.

I barely remember their home. My eyes shoot daggers toward the bed in the living room as soon as we walk in, hyper-focused on this old sleeping man whom I'm aware hates everyone who looks like me. There is a perception of death doulas as full of lavender and lace, but I'm not. I'm more lapis lazuli and lamé. People think that we are angels because of the work we do, but my sisters and ex-boyfriends would laugh in your face at the suggestion that I'm an angel. If you don't fuck with me, I don't fuck with you. Plain and simple. I'll send love your way, but from afar. I'm still human.

In the kitchen I sit at the table near the window and try not to fume. They offer me tea, which I decline. I'm here to do a job, after all, and get out. There is a tablecloth with lemons printed on it and a bowl of aging fruit in the center, littered with random papers, note-pads, and pill bottles. This table could fit in any home where some-one is seriously ill and dying: everyone handling tasks, forgetting to eat. John, dressed like his brother's twin but in a white button-down shirt, is happy to see me and offers an equally empty apology. He knows what they have done is reprehensible. They have invited me into a space that is violent to me and serves their own good without concern for mine. They've either never heard of consent or don't care. This is whiteness at its most opportunistic.

I try to get straight to the point so I can get out of hell's kitchen. They tell me that the doctor is fine giving Jack additional medica-tion. But he is already at a high dosage of opiates, and Andrew is concerned about addiction. I talk them through a cost-benefit risk analysis—risk of addiction (very low) versus further pain (high), complications versus comfort. The hospice nurse has just arrived, and I wonder if she has some info that I haven't heard yet.

After Andrew gets permission from Jack for the hospice nurse to talk to me, she explains that Jack has an obstruction in his bowels that might be causing him pain. I watch silently as she palpates his abdomen. He barely winces. She moves her hands and pushes down harder. No grimace, no moan. She asks how he is doing. He says he is fine, but then immediately asks when he will get his opiates. This language is unusual to me. Most people would usually just call it "medicine."

The hospice nurse asks about his level of pain and Jack immediately says it's at a nine out of ten. I'm surprised, because it certainly doesn't look like the racist is in pain. However, a person's subjective experience of pain is not for another to judge. Pain is as it is reported. Disbelieving reported pain is one of the main factors contributing to Black people's lack of access to pain management and to Black maternal mortality. When someone says they are in pain, emotional or physical, believe them. I choose to believe him.

The nurse busies herself preparing Jack's transdermal pain patches and cleaning his skin to attach them to his abdomen. I avert my eyes to offer some privacy but inside, I wish he were on display like the Hottentot Venus. While I only agreed to talk to his sons, I've already agreed to help, so I commit to doing my job as thoroughly as possible. Against my better judgment, this means talking to Jack. When the nurse is done, she heads into the kitchen with Jack's sons to give us some privacy. I hear them start to whisper.

Jack's eyes are bloodshot and his cheeks are ruddy from years of alcoholism and illness. Deep brown and purple liver spots color his body and his lips are cracked, chapped, and a little bluish. I take a deep breath. "Do you know why I'm here?"

He glances at me with disdain, then looks away. "Yes, but I don't know what you think you'll be able to do for me." His voice sounds like a lifetime of whiskey and cigarettes. "They said you were going to make sure I got my opiates. But I didn't realize you were a colored girl." For a man with red and purple spots, blue lips, and white hair, he's got some nerve calling *me* colored. I'm a deep chocolate brown everywhere, including where the sun don't shine. Realizing that at eighty-eight years old, this is likely the language and terminology he is most accustomed to, I'm trying to be understanding and compassionate. But it still fucking pisses me off. He knows better. He must.

"Yes. I am Black. And that's got nothing to do with how I do my job, which has nothing to do with whether or not you get the medicine. I'm not a doctor and the nurse just gave you a patch."

"Then what are you doing in my house?"

Breathe, Alua. Fix your face, Alua. I'm trying to appear calm on the outside, but inside I'm fighting him. "Your sons and nurse tell me that you're in pain. I'm sorry about that." This is a lie. In reality I wish he were getting stabbed by a million needles in his eyeballs while kicked in the kneecaps by donkeys. "They also tell me that you're dying. Are you thinking much about that?"

He scoffs. "What do you think? I can't go anywhere, and I can't do anything. All day long I lay here doing jack shit but thinking that I'm going to die. It's something everyone has to do at some point, and I guess it's just my turn. But you should already understand that." He enunciates every word as though I'm five years old. He hasn't looked back at me.

Breathe, Alua. Fix your face, Alua. "I do understand that, but I also understand that knowing that you're dying can come with a lot of emotions, and some of them are unpleasant. Are you having any of those?"

"What is this navel-gazing bullshit? I don't want to think about the fact that I am dying. I don't want you asking me anything about death. I don't want to talk about it. And I don't want to talk to you. I just want my opiates." *There's that word again.* "If you can't get them for me, then get the fuck out of my house." Spittle flies out of his hateful mouth along with his hateful words, as he finally turns to look at me full-on.

Breathe, Alua. Fix your face, Alua. I take another deep breath and consider if I should engage. This is a weighing act every Black person I know does when interfacing with white America. I want to curse him out and tell him that I hope he gags on a bag of dicks on his joyride to the underworld. But I also want to preserve my internal peace, which this man is threatening to disrupt. If I leave, have I let him win? If I stay and engage, angry and vengeful, have I let him win? He won't win. Not today, Satan.

What is happening with Jack and his desire for opiates is clear to me. He is in deep emotional, psychic, and existential pain. He doesn't want to be around for his dying. Plus, he is hateful. That hurts him more than it will ever hurt me. It is eating him alive from the inside. Given his bowel obstruction, he is literally full of shit.

Without answering him, I head back into the kitchen to Andrew and John, who sit at the table looking like lost congressional aides. I've gotten all of the information I need and taken all the abuse I have capacity for. Andrew and John stand suddenly and look at me in alarm. I guess I haven't adequately fixed my face.

"What happened?!" John asks, aghast.

My words careen out of my mouth as fast as I can speak them so I can leave. "Your father is a hateful, angry, and scared man. I believe he is clear he is dying but does not want to be around for the process. You said he was addicted to opiates when he came back from the Korean War? Right?"

They both look at me, dumbfounded.

"Right??" I ask again with force, and they nod fast. "He likely medicated the pain from the war with his opiates then and is probably medicating the pain of facing his death now. He keeps asking for 'opiates' rather than pain medication. And I think he knows he has to report that he is in pain in order to get his opiates." I pause. "Anything else?" I grab my bag, sitting next to the fruit bowl on the table. A dozen fruit flies scatter away.

I'm done and I'm angry. I'm angry with them for asking Black-ass me to come, knowing that their father hates people with my skin. I am angry at this country. But I am angriest with myself for agreeing to do it anyway.

"So should we give him the medication? Won't he get addicted?" Andrew asks.

I throw up my hands. "He's dying anyway. I can't tell you what to do. But I've told you what I think. And now I'm ready to leave. Out of the *front door*."

I cry frustrated tears on the drive home. I hate the duplicity with which Jack's sons brought me into his space and I'm angry at myself for softening my boundaries. Just because I am a helper does not mean that I put myself in any ole situation when I can help. Sometimes it causes me more harm than good. Before being confronted with a racist client, I would have told you that I'd never do it. But I have just done it. I wonder if I have unconsciously made myself small to make white people comfortable, yet again.

I quickly shake my head and am reminded to honor the holiness of my no. It is just as powerful as my yes. Jack forces me to find my edges and boundaries in this work that means so much to me. This is a major step for anyone who chooses death work.

Andrew's wife calls me while I'm on the road. I clear my throat and adjust my voice so she can't hear my pain. It sickens me when white people know that they've caused me pain because of my race. She has spoken to her husband and her voice drips with apology about what her father-in-law said to me and who he is. She also tells me that Andrew and John have agreed to give Jack additional pain medication and have communicated it to him. Upon hearing the news that I was able to help give him what he wanted, racist, angry Jack sings my Black praises. He calls me an angel and a "sweet girl." How quickly I turned from someone not worthy to be in his house to someone to celebrate when he got what he wanted from me. Typical.

I never saw Jack again. And I've never accepted another client whose beliefs included hate. I won't do that to myself again.

Even as I despised Jack and the way he treated me, I could see how much he was loved. To me, Jack was a monster. My stomach turned thinking about how much power he wielded in the military and what he did with it. But to others, he was a father, a grandfather, a fellow soldier, a friend, and—most important—a human being. His legacy is much greater than his hatred of Black people, but this is the Jack that I met. Even with my personal animus toward him, choosing to hold Jack only in his hatred diminishes the totality of who he was as a human—his light and his darkness. And I don't believe in throwing humans away. Anger and compassion don't mix. Compassion calls me to forgive him.

I am reluctant to answer that call, but I do not know his whole story, his history, his glowing qualities, the loving words people said at his funeral, and the deep grief they felt when he was gone. I do know that people who hurt us eventually die, and sometimes the grief is convoluted when we loved them despite their worst parts.

As I seek to understand these contradictions, I ask myself: When have I been guilty of loving someone who might have been hurting others? The capacity to hurt others, after all, is as human as the capacity to be hurt. Each of us, at some point in our lives, has found ourselves struggling with this complicated love.

Speaking of which.

Michael Jackson was my first crush. He was my first inspiration, my first idol. He was also my first impactful death. Sometimes it feels like I've never felt a love as pure as my childhood love of the man they called the King of Pop.

Michael Jackson could do everything. He floated above the ground, which lit up when he touched it. His melodies were pure, as was his voice, and he transmitted love. He came to us from everywhere— into our living rooms on our television sets, gliding across stages, in malls, on T-shirts, and blasting joyfully out of passing cars. He seemed to be made of magic and he sprinkled it everywhere he went.

He danced and his moves entranced me. At five years old, I was glued to the television watching the "Thriller" video—scared and exhilarated, while Bozoma hid under the table. My sisters and I performed dance shows for our parents' friends to the *Bad* album. I tried to learn the fight scene in "Beat It" to toughen up my nonviolent self—turns out, didn't work. The only time I got into a fight as a child, I cried and asked the boy why he hit me. I wanted to understand him.

As I grew up, Michael Jackson came with me. I remember Ahoba yelling at me from the bottom of the stairs in 1992 to get off the phone because I was missing the beginning of the worldwide premiere of the "Remember the Time" video. I had to sneak to watch his "In the Closet" video—deemed too sexy by my conservative Christian parents—and snaked my head back and forth, imitating the dance moves from "Black or White." When Bozoma went away to Wesleyan in 1999, I had the radio deejay dedicate "You Are Not Alone" to her, saddened about how lonely she must have been without us. Sometimes I wonder if my love of musicians originated with him.

The first time I heard abuse allegations against Michael Jackson, in 1993, I was fifteen years old. My first thought was, *Well, this must be a mistake. Or a misunderstanding. He's a celebrity.* Or so I reasoned. These types of things happened all the time. I was in too deep, too blinded by my adoration, to consider the possibility. I don't believe the thought that the allegations were true flitted across my mind for a second. When the case was settled, I shrugged with relief. *Poor Michael,* I thought. The media were so cruel to him.

It was only years later, when I watched him dangle his baby Blanket off a balcony above the waiting heads of paparazzi, that I felt an uneasy something sitting in my gut. As the allegations mounted, I grew more desperate for them not to be true. The ugliness was too much; the implications were too shattering. I stuck my head in the sand. I wanted to preserve my image of my idol. It was difficult to shed my defensive sense of Michael as a saint who needed my protection. No one had ever lived under that intense microscope in the history of humankind. He was globally famous in a way that was hard to comprehend. Long before Chiang Mai, Thailand, was a popular travel destination, I'd had a fruit vendor lick his finger and rub it on my skin to show me that if I showered more often, my skin color would come off. *Like Michael Jackson,* he added helpfully. (Surprising only him, my skin did not change color.)

Anyone would suffer under a spotlight that bright. And genius is usually linked with a touch of madness, right? Could he be anything other than perfect? It took me years to reckon with what these allegations may have meant, both to the idea I held of him in my heart and the families that were impacted.

The day Michael Jackson died, I was in my office at Legal Aid, working on an affidavit of support for a domestic violence restraining order for one of my clients. We had an appointment the next day for her to sign the documents and file them. My secretary, Veronica, rushed in my always-open office door.

She launched right in. "Did you hear?"

"Hear what?" I finished typing my sentence before fully turning my attention to her.

"They are saying that Michael Jackson has died." She whispered it like a secret.

"Michael Jackson who?" I asked incredulously, trying to make sense of what she had just said. "Who's saying that?"

She fiddled with her pearl necklace. "It's all over TMZ."

I scoffed. The source wasn't credible to me and as such, neither was the news.

"We can't trust them," I said. "That's not true. Farrah Fawcett already died today." As though two celebrities couldn't die the same day. I didn't want to believe it, so I turned back to my computer. Sheepishly, Veronica left my office. I sat at my desk unable to work, trying to make sense of the possibility that my childhood idol could have died. He didn't. He couldn't. He was supposed to be immortal.

Slowly, it became real. As I spoke one by one with my family members and friends who had called to check up on me because they all knew of my love for him, they corroborated the impossible. Michael Joseph Jackson, the man whom I thought I would marry when I was eight years old, the man who created the soundtrack to my childhood and adolescence, the man I idolized for his expression and artistry, and the man I'd watched in horror as he fell publicly from grace, was, in fact, dead. The numbness of this inconceivable truth pinned me to my desk chair.

Suddenly, I needed to get out of the office. I needed to feel that joyous feeling of "The Way You Make Me Feel." With a quick good-bye to Veronica and an affidavit of support left unfinished, I jumped into my Jeep in the parking lot. The sound system wasn't great, but the speakers I'd upgraded the month before and the bass tube I put in the back helped. The auxiliary cable was already plugged into my hot-pink iPod Shuffle but the battery was dead. Out of frustration, I shook the iPod and noticed the butterfly sticker on the back. The melody for the song "Butterflies" popped in my head.

NOT MICHAEL JACKSON.

I rolled down the window and started the car, in a rush to get home. I needed to hear my favorite songs, although it would have been impossible to choose. All were my favorite and none were adequate for the gravity of that moment. Then, waiting for the stoplight to change in mid-city Los Angeles, I heard faint music. Someone was playing "Billie Jean" loudly from their parked car in front of the strip mall to my right. My heart surged. I kept driving. As the light changed and I drove west on Washington Boulevard toward my home, I saw people gathered in a post office parking lot on the corner of Washington and Crenshaw. Mixed melodies rang out. All Michael Jackson tunes. I slammed on the brakes and made a sharp left to join the crowd. I didn't know what they were doing, but I wanted to be a part of it. Puzzlingly, grief longs both for solitude and community. Grief itself is a puzzle.

As I rolled through the parking lot, songs blared from car stereos. "Rock with You." I wanted to own his sparkly jumpsuit in this video. "PYT"—somewhat of a theme song for me, as I tended to date people younger than me. "Man in the Mirror" regularly reminds me that all change starts within. People milled about. No one was going in or out of the post office and a few people in post office uniforms were among them. Seems they had simply found themselves there in a shared moment of grief and joined like I was doing. I parked my car in the first spot I could find. A man parked next to me sat with the driver side door of his car open and his head in his hands.

A reporter on his car radio was reporting from the hospital where Michael Jackson's body had been taken. The man looked up as I approached. Shaking his head, he took off his baseball cap and revealed a small gray fade in need of a cut. All he said was "Michael Jackson, man." He paused. "Michael Jackson." His eyes were wet and bloodshot. The sight of this older Black man sitting in his green sedan crying about Michael Jackson's death finally broke me.

"Same," I responded through my own belated tears. "Same." I wept, for the loss of my childhood idol, the loss of my innocence about our safety from death, and for anyone who survived molestation who was triggered by his glorification in the news.

Till the sun went down on the day Michael Jackson died, I stayed in that parking lot, dancing, singing, crying, and witnessing the shared grief of perfect strangers for a man whose legacy, for better and worse, was larger than a single life.

Some people leave complex legacies—meadows teeming with beautiful wildflowers and lethal toxins. We all do, in various ratios. And we truly have no idea how we or the landscape will transform in the ages to come. The Michael Jackson I loved is long since gone, but what he created remains and it is still alive within me. It will be with me until my death, and that I cannot deny. Why do we reduce people to the worst thing they've done? Or the best? When does someone stop being a father and become only an adulterer?

With people we love, we choose to remember them mostly in their magic. This is why some say that grief is the price we pay for love. But it is much more complicated than that. We freely grieve the things we love and will miss. It's that way with all of us and I see it often in my work. I am still attached to Michael Jackson's magic, despite all that happened afterward. While that creates complex layers to our grief, it does not lessen it. He was a whole human with stories, pains, and joys we will never know about that people who did know him well will intensely grieve. We cannot deny them that. I bet Andrew and John felt something similar about their racist father.

It is okay to mourn people in all their complexity, to honor their light, acknowledge their darkness, to accept the message in spite of the messenger. The very worst of us will still probably be missed by *some*one when they're gone. Appreciated by someone. Loved by someone. Remembered fondly by someone for something. This is the full capacity of humanity at work.

Chapter 14

People Who Need People

I arrived at the Denver International Airport (DIA) in September 2012 after leaving Portland and Pascha. I was harried, haggard, bruised, and uncertain. Despite my recent medical leave of absence, I didn't feel free—just cut loose and drifting.

I had no return ticket back to my home in L.A., and my next stop was unknown. I'd flown into DIA a hundred times, often coming from some faraway place to visit my parents, who still lived in Colorado for most of my young adulthood. This time, I was visiting Kristin, whose serendipitous phone call had rescued me from the brink of collapse in Portland.

Kristin and I met through a study group of close friends during my first year in law school. We formed a quick bond. Rachel MacGuire, Jenni Cohen, Kristin Bowers Tompkins, and Jess Curtis remain the smartest and most hysterically crass women I've ever met. When Kristin and her law school boyfriend broke up, we baked a carrot cake and ate the whole thing in one sitting. At Jess's bachelorette party, we got kicked out of an Irish pub when a woman at the next table tried to insult me by calling me fat. All five feet four inches of Kristin (and five feet three inches of Rachel) jumped over the table in a flash to kick her ass, light-up penis headbands still on their heads. At Jess's wedding, we all dove into the pool in our bridesmaid's dresses, much to the horror of the other guests. We celebrated when Kristin called off her wedding, by wearing black veils, in Santa Fe, New Mexico, and that night I admitted quietly for the first time that I did not want to be married either. When her father died, I cried with her.

At DIA, my large backpack arrived on the carousel with an open zipper. Regardless, I bounced out of the terminal excited to see my friend and to be on to my next adventure. She looked worried as she helped me load my backpack into the trunk. "You're so skinny," she said, an observation that only my mother, sisters, and very best friends are allowed to make to me out of concern for my health.

"Thanks? I'm okay!" I responded. Kristin isn't the type to congratulate you on weight loss, so she knew something was up. I was eager to convince her that I was not as ill as I was.

Unsmiling and hesitant, she gave me a quick nod and we pulled off. We made small talk about my flight and my last adventure in Portland with Pascha. She was unsurprised that I flew to meet a man I'd known for a few hours, but quite surprised that we didn't fall in love as I've done time and again.

An hour later, we arrived at Kristin's home and I settled into her spare room. She and her partner, Luke, had recently returned to Denver after a two-year trip visiting national parks and sleeping in a Suburban they'd outfitted for the trip. The spare room held a desk full of papers, a mattress pad they'd named Paco, and camping gear on the floor. They'd set out a mountain of comforters for me.

"It's all we've got for now," she said unapologetically. Kristin moved through the world with little apology, and I admired that about her. I wanted some of that for myself.

While Kristin and I chatted excitedly in the small room, I started to settle in, unpacking my half-open bag. Then I noticed one of the fancy Camper shoes I'd bought for my trip was missing, and burst into tears. I'd only packed a couple of pairs of shoes—sandals in case I went somewhere warm, running shoes to keep up my already-frayed mental health with my daily run. I'd been living on my disability income only, plus the meager savings I'd amassed from my part-time job at Legal Aid, and $225 for a new pair was a huge splurge.

I was inconsolable. Depression had clouded my sense of proportion: small things felt like big things and big things were simply insurmountable. This felt like a very big thing, and I was clearly crying about more than a shoe. Kristin listened patiently with her hand on my back as I tried to explain my disproportionate reaction. Portland with Pascha had been a mess, and I didn't know what I was doing or where I was going next during my leave. I'd tried so hard to keep up the appearance that I could handle traveling in the midst of my illness, but one missing shoe shattered the facade.

I was fatigued from the two-hour flight, but only because I was otherwise exhausted. Depression itself is exhausting. It lies heavy on the body like a wet velvet cloak, muting your connection to the outside world. Paco, the sleeping pad on the floor, beckoned. Kristin hesitated at the door before leaving. "You sure you're okay?" She'd never seen me like this before. Nobody had. I nodded feebly, aware that whatever pretense I was clinging to had slipped. She closed the door and I cried again out of shame.

In the morning, light flooded the little room. Colorado is famous for its three hundred days of sunshine. I hoped it could make me feel happy and bright again, but the single shoe lying at the edge of my backpack reminded me of what an utter disappointment I was. I got out of bed, but was unsure how to act.

"Hey y'all!" I called into the kitchen from the hallway.

"Hey you! How'd you sleep?" Kristin asked.

I tried my hand at faking joy. "Great! I love how much light the room gets!" In reality I had tossed and turned, angry at myself for spending so much money on shoes and for being careless enough to bring them with me.

Kristin started walking toward me and I wanted to run, afraid she wanted to talk about the night before. I hid my head because I didn't want her to see my puffy eyes. Instead, she offered a hoodie from Luke's closet—my backpack wasn't big enough for such items of comfort. I love wearing a man's sweatshirt because it feels like a hug from a man, and at this point, I needed all the hugs I could get. I followed her into her closet to get the white Quiksilver hoodie, which became a second skin during my stay. Standing in the closet, I took off my shirt to add to the laundry, and Kristin gasped. Her eyes made it clear that my body resembled how I felt. Like a hollow shell with little light or life left inside.

In a year, I'd lost about forty pounds without noticing. Even though my baby fat came off naturally through adulthood, my concern for how my belly lay over my waistband, where my legs rubbed together, or my back rolls touched each other never fully abated. When depression hit, my internalized fatphobia disappeared. I was too busy trying to make it through each day. My athletic, hourglass figure started to look more like a pencil. My breasts deflated and my hips lost their curves. Skeletal dents emerged in my shoulders, and my ribs were visible in both my chest and my back. My cheekbones became even sharper and my collarbone jutted out of my chest. I was gaunt. My body was a ghost of itself.

"Alua," whispered Kristin. "You gotta eat. Please. Let me make you breakfast."

"Oh, don't worry about it!" I responded, still faking joy. "I'll figure something out when you go to work." This was a lie. The idea of making a meal completely overwhelmed me, and Kristin sniffed me out, unwilling to leave me to my own devices. "I'm gonna make you something. What do you want?"

"No, please don't do that! I'm fine," I insisted.

She didn't let up. "It won't be anything big," she replied. "Just something for you to nibble when you get hungry."

"Don't, okay? Just don't." I rolled my eyes, wishing she'd leave it alone, but Kristin is gloriously stubborn in the direction of what she believes is good. She walked back to the kitchen.

"Why don't you go take a shower? I'll be gone by the time you finish and you can eat in peace."

I walked to the bathroom, seething. *How dare she try to force me to do something I don't want to do?* Looking at my body in the mirror, however, I understood. I saw the bones and sagging flesh. I was embarrassed. I cursed her out loud in the shower for knowing me so well. Maybe I shouldn't have come to Colorado to stay with her after all. I could still leave and go someplace where I could continue to hide from the prying eyes of people who loved me. Damn them and their worries. I was fine.

Kristin left a plate on the counter with an egg-and-cheese sandwich on an English muffin and some cut up strawberries. A bottle of hot sauce sat on the right. To the left of the plate was a note held down by an apple. The note read:

> *8:30am: Breakfast! Here's your sandwich. Sorry can't remember*
>   *if you like hot sauce or not.*
> *10:30am: Snack! Raid the pantry :)*
> *1pm: Lunch—there's tuna fish on the second shelf in the fridge*
>   *and two pieces of bread. There are baby carrots in the crisper*
>   *and kettle chips in the pantry.*
> *3pm: Another snack! Have this apple with peanut butter.*
> *5pm: I'll order pizza for dinner!!*
> *Have a great day! I'll check on you. PLEASE PLEASE EAT.*

I paced back and forth in the blue and white kitchen and debated eating. To eat would mean that I accepted her support. To *not* eat would be to reject it, and also waste food. Despite being African, growing up, we'd been taught to think of all the starving children in America. I couldn't do that to them. I ate the sandwich, begrudgingly. If she could see through my strong-woman exterior, could others? Had they been able to tell that I was suffering? That idea alone caused me more embarrassment.

Growing up in my family, my sisters and I learned to prioritize strength and resilience; as far as I was concerned, vulnerability was not a virtue.

Sitting there chewing and stewing, I was surprised to find this hardness within me. Where had it come from? I didn't extend it to others. As a Legal Aid attorney, offering support to those who needed it was the crux of my work. I had never thought any less of my clients who suffered violence at the hands of their partners. I had not judged those who did not have enough money for food. I'd inherently understood that my clients were not at fault for their situations. Classism, racism, broken systems, and childhood traumas had led them there. And even if they had a hand in it, they were still worthy of having someone care enough to help them out.

And yet depression felt like a personal failure on my part, as though I was not strong enough to keep myself happy and healthy. I had failed the ultimate test. I had not stayed "strong."

Being "strong" is built into my genetic makeup. My mother is an absolute pillar. She stayed at home taking care of me and my sisters while we traveled, spreading the word of God until my father lost his job in Colorado Springs. Without an advanced formal education, her option was to work the late shift at a steel plant in the Springs. Sometimes she'd come home around 11 P.M. with burns on her forearms and still wake up early to make sure we had breakfast and our school projects were in order. She stayed up all night to pack for flights, cooked feasts for our friends for any small reason or none at all, and walked thirteen miles just because she could. You rarely catch her napping, and she is proud of this fact.

African women have long been the backbones of their families, which has carried over into African American cultural norms. Black women are expected to carry the weight of the family and the world while doing it with grace. The R & B group Destiny's Child did us no favors with their song "Independent Woman," an anthem for women that screams "I depend on me!" I certainly still sing it at the top of my lungs, but it's fucking absurd. No offense to Queen Beyoncé who does no wrong, but they (and society) sold us a raw deal.

What is so wrong with needing someone? Have we failed as women if we do? Are we no longer worthy of love?

On the contrary, I was receiving a lot of love from Kristin. She'd opened her home for me to share with her and her partner, whom I barely knew. She'd offered me comfortable clothing for my stay. She had made me meals. She'd even listened as I cried uncontrollably about my missing shoe. My vulnerability seemed to be uncovering the depth of the love that she had for me.

When I let Kristin see me, I finally let a part of me die that had been keeping love at bay. I'd been so "strong" that I hadn't allowed anyone to take care of me outside of childhood. "I got it" and "I'm good" had become mantras that led to burnout at work and the absence of real intimacy. But I wanted a gentle life. A tender life. A lush life. A soft life. Not one that required me to be strong. To do that, I needed to surrender to help.

I scowled at Kristin's breakfast sandwich while I ate it. Each bite I took was an admission of my inability to care for myself properly. It went down my throat like sandpaper.

Some of us go our entire lives without surrendering to help. Many of my clients are self-made islands by the time I get to meet them. Sometimes as a death doula I get to be the message in the bottle that washes ashore, telling them it's never too late to extend a hand into that empty space before you, daring to ask for help.

Dying is the most intimate act we will undertake. It requires us to be intimate with ourselves, our bodies, our lives, and with the present moment—to reveal the parts we believe are difficult to love, the face beneath the mask we wear for the outside world, and the squishy parts that bear wounds and form scars. Everything else is a show. To be helped is to die a small death of the ego. To allow love in is an invitation to allow our messy human glory to take front stage, and let love pour into those places that have been beaten down by the ego and the outside world.

That happened with my client Claudia. She calls me to talk about a potential end of life planning session after a pulmonary embolism lands her in the hospital for three weeks. At fifty-seven, she is shook that the blood clot could have ended her life. Both emotionally and practically, she is not ready. Her death would have been a sudden one.

When someone dies suddenly, we often say their death was un-expected, as though we all cannot expect that death will come one day. Unless we are struck dead when in perfect health, most of us will wind up feeble and weak. Most often it comes far sooner than we are ready for. Either a diagnosis lands out of the blue, or a disease progresses much faster than we expected. Our bodies are fragile. It only takes a nick of a rusty blade or a faulty heart valve to turn a strapping twenty-one-year-old into a corpse. Everyone old enough to have a credit card or a driver's license should be planning for their death. Some consider it a gift to know that their lives are ending as a result of disease; it gives them the opportunity to get acquainted. Death comes either as a friend or a stranger. It is up to us to decide.

"Isn't it too early to be talking to a death doula? I mean, I don't think I'm gonna die soon," says *literally everyone* except for the very elderly.

"Depends," I usually reply, tongue firmly in cheek. "When is too early to start planning for something you know one day is gonna happen, but could happen tomorrow?"

"Well, when you put it that way, I guess I should start planning now." Works every time.

With Claudia, we've already established a good rapport, as she's asked a million questions about what death doulas do and has deter-mined it's a match for her needs. Since she'd had a lengthy hospital stay after her pulmonary embolism, Claudia understands the neces-sity of support. Someone had to take care of her dogs, water her plants, handle her bills, collect her mail, throw out food in her fridge, and so on. She got a taste of what happens to everybody eventually. After our deaths, someone else will rifle through every aspect of our lives, closing accounts and throwing away most of the physical evidence that we lived. Claudia's come to grips with this and is ready to prepare.

She and I decide to complete a comprehensive end of life planning document to get all her affairs in order. We meet in person for the three-hour session. She's brown-skinned, Nicaraguan, plump, short, and jolly, with a hug that feels like climbing into a familiar bathtub, especially because I have to bend down to embrace her. Her home is warm, covered in plants, and decorated in yellows and browns with a big burnt-sienna sectional by the window facing the fireplace, which houses two dog beds for her elderly animals. The chocolate Labradors barely register my presence when I arrive. The colors also match her bouncy, curly bob haircut with a few flecks of gray showing at the roots. There are orange candles burning, which makes her house smell like cloves and Christmas, even though it is April. She brings me a cup of herbal tea and I settle into the long end of the couch while Claudia takes a spot in the nook.

We chat quickly about the packet I've brought her—the advance planning document, a pencil, and some business cards. Once the document is completed—in pencil, as it's intended to be a living document and thus plenty subject to change—it will be legally binding. She is taken aback by its heft. Most people are surprised by the amount of work it takes to prepare for death. It helps to have a guide on the path.

End of life planning looks different for each person, to meet their unique needs. But some areas are necessary for everyone. Advance directives are a smart place to start.

Choosing a healthcare proxy is the most important decision to make.

Claudia and I open up the document and begin. First up: healthcare decision-making. I describe what a healthcare decision-maker does and explain the permissions we grant them when we are incapacitated. Called a healthcare agent, a healthcare proxy, or a medical surrogate (depending on the location and entity), this is the person who will make decisions when it is deemed that someone is incapable of making them on their own. This is a position of deep trust and mutual respect. This person might hold life in their hands.

The first time I ask Claudia whom she would like to make decisions for her, she gets squirmy and asks to take a break before we've even properly started. I hear her sighing and rummaging through things in the other room. When she returns with nothing in her hands to show for it, I ask again. Flipping forward and squinting at the pages ahead, she asks if we can skip this part. Making a mental note of her discomfort, I agree to move on to Section 2, on life support, and suggest we circle back.

Almost three hours later, she's named a caregiver for her dogs, detailed her desires for life-sustaining treatment, catalogued her passwords, and promised (tomorrow, she says!) to contact the lawyer who helped her draft her will. We've listed her bank and retirement accounts, written down desires for her body disposition, and made a few notes about what she wants at her service—daffodils everywhere, and everyone *must* cry, she adds, to lighten the mood. I've also made a few notes to remind me of the sections we'll have to revisit in the follow-up meeting.

Throughout most of the consultation, Claudia is indefatigable. She even sails through the life support conversation, which typically unnerves people. I have yet to meet anyone who is thrilled at the thought of their bodies lying unresponsive and on the brink of death on a table, kept alive by machines. One question to contemplate while planning for the end of life is "What condition of living is worse than dying?" I ask this question in end of life planning sessions to help clients make value-based decisions about life support treatment. Rather than asking a client for a blanket yes or no answer to the desire to have an intervening treatment to hold off an impend-ing death, I find it's useful to help them tease out the "why" of the decisions. It is impossible to think of the millions of scenarios that could lead to a need for life support from our current vantage point. The "what if" game can run rampant. "What if I am ninety-five?" "What if I'm pregnant and in a coma?" "What if I have only one eye and a quarter of a foot?" We can narrow down our desires using our values as the foundation. This allows our loved ones who are tasked with carrying out our decisions to make an informed choice about life support.

In response to the question about values, many say they do not want to be a burden on their loved ones. A deeper exploration into this statement sometimes reflects a value system based on time or money—they do not want their loved ones to have to spend a lot of time and money to keep them alive. But what is the monetary value of a life? How much time is okay to spend caring for someone who is loved? For curiosity's sake I often ask for clarity how much a client thinks their life is worth, as though their loved ones will turn off the machines as soon as the credit cards have to come out or they want to go to a dinner. I have yet to meet a beloved family member who made a decision about ending life support treatment based solely upon how much it cost or how much time it takes. While treatments at the end of life are ludicrously expensive, decisions to end life sup-port are often based on knowing that a loved one would not want to live hooked up to a machine.

Many others say they want to be able to communicate as a condi-tion of extending life support but levels of communication can vary greatly. It's hard for many people to imagine when healthy and able-bodied, however. It reeks of ableism. People with diseases where motor neurons in the brain and spinal cord break down have found inventive ways to communicate, although they might experience slurred speech or lose the ability to speak altogether. Hand gestures, facial expressions, and even some high-tech devices support them in communication.

For some reason, it was easier for Claudia to handle that part of the planning than it was to name who should make her decisions for her if she can't.

"Is there someone in your life you trust to make your decisions for you in the event that you can't?" I ask for the third time.

"No," says Claudia. It's a one-word sentence. But something isn't adding up, so carefully I push further.

"What about your siblings?" I know Claudia is the oldest of five and helped take care of her younger siblings when they were all growing up in Nicaragua. After her move to the US, she continued to send money home to care for her family. Eventually, she was able to help a few of them move to the States and they rely on her for financial and child-rearing support. I'm surprised she doesn't name one of them. She just shakes her head.

"Alright," I say, keeping my voice even, despite my growing curiosity. "What about the friends who show up for you when you need them?"

Claudia thinks for a moment and shakes her head again. Her mantel is full of snapshots of family outings, birthday parties, nights on the town with friends, and children. Vacations, weddings, graduations. This clearly isn't a woman who lives in solitude. Her warmth makes me think that she is well-liked, unless she hides her ugly side well. There is something I am missing.

"What about the person who walked your dog and watered your plants when you were in the hospital?"

"I paid someone," she responds, avoiding eye contact. When I catch her eyes, they are wet and she wipes away a tear before it smudges her mascara.

Claudia explains that she has a lot of friends but she is the one that people call when they are in need. She drops her plans and her priorities to help others. When she was in the hospital, many asked what they could do to help, but she repeated that she had it all taken care of. The balance of giving and receiving is so off in her life that she no longer knows how to receive care. She's grown toxically self-reliant and believes that others won't come to her aid when she needs them. It's become a self-fulfilling prophecy.

This toxic self-reliance often rears its head near the deathbed. So often in end of life planning conversations, clients who have been fiercely independent their whole lives will make gruff declarations like "If I can't wipe my own ass, take me out back and shoot me!" These clients often ascribe to a version of the quintessential American myth: they came from "nothing" and made "something" of themselves without relying upon anyone. They regale me with stories about how they've pulled themselves up by their bootstraps. These stories overlook the privilege they relied upon, or the dozens of people who handed them a sandwich when they were hungry, let them pay rent a couple of days late, or even let them use the bathroom at the coffee shop.

To exist in a society means to live with others. And no person, despite what they think, is an island. In this modern age, dying happens in community. It takes doctors, nurses, caregivers, food prep, childcare; the list goes on.

Most of us will die from disease. This means a slow descent into helplessness. We're all going to need someone eventually. Even a client's request to "take me out back and shoot me" would require the assistance of another person. Our lives in their conception are a collaboration. Sperm meets egg.

I understand how hard it is to turn ourselves over to someone else: to trust another with our hearts, fears, dark, shadowy parts, and to also trust that we will be taken care of and still be loved. It's hard to surrender into being vulnerable. Claudia has built a fortress around herself from fear of being disappointed by people who won't show up for her like she shows up for them. In this way, she is setting herself up for others not to support her in her death either. She literally cannot think of one person whom she can trust to make her deci- sions in case of serious illness or at her death. She only trusts herself because she hasn't trusted anyone *with* herself.

After a decent cry with her curly hair bouncing along with her shoulders, Claudia says that she will talk to her younger sister about her hospital stay and use it as a segue to talk about death. Of her siblings, this sister would be most likely to respect her wishes and do what Claudia wants even if she wouldn't want it herself. The very idea of the conversation makes Claudia writhe some more. It's hard to need when we have let others need us instead. But we all need to get over ourselves and need someone, already.

I'm sad for Claudia. But I'm also sad for the thousands of times I haven't let others care for me. I have not given them the oppor- tunity to love me by caring for me and have blocked the energetic cycle of abundance by refusing their gift of care. Society tells us that the epitome of womanhood is to be selfless. To give and give until the patriarchy has taken all, and we can be docile and con- trolled. We are not to have any needs. A bottomless well without the groundwater to fill it back up. Who is supposed to fill us back up? How are we supposed to learn how to receive it?

Claudia helps me see that my lack of willingness to let anyone help me made me into an island. A supposed lone wolf, where it had become damn near impossible for me to let someone help me carry my groceries, let alone take care of me in my most vulnerable moments.

The negative messaging around neediness comes from everywhere: I've heard people complain about how their needy partners and home- girls complain about that one friend who calls too often. Yet there have been many times I needed a long hug from a friend, to cry with one of my sisters, or to spend some time with my man. Am I "needy"? What's so bad about having needs? Or are these basic human requests? I think of how I choked on voicing my needs whenever my mom or friends called, asking if I was alright. I shrank myself to avoid feeling like a burden and measured my strength by how much pain I could endure on my own.

One of my deepest core desires is to be loved and appreciated. I fulfill it by taking care of others in my classic ride-or-die way—I ride *and* die. Sitting with Claudia, I could see how that could impact me in my own dying, if I never hit rock bottom enough to get vulnerable. I struggled to accept help until I had absolutely no choice.

Chapter 15

Breaking Open

My days in Colorado with Kristin mostly rolled into each other. Each morning, she left a menu, and Luke told me his activities for the day in case I wanted to join him. I usually declined unless he was going for a bike ride, since he shared my love of bikes, and he'd cleaned up an old red Schwinn ten-speed for me to use. My days were filled with people-watching through the living room window, long, lazy bike rides, and wondering why I still felt paralyzed. I found no answers, and then I thought about an old fling, Joshua, who used to have access to psychedelic drugs. Maybe they could help me shake this. At the very least it would be an interesting way to spend the afternoon. I called him.

My use of psychedelics up until that point had mostly been for healing purposes with the occasional recreational use during Halloween in college (horrifying choice) and at the Burning Man festival (a good choice, then and always). My experiences with LSD, psilocybin, ayahuasca, ketamine, and DMT have taught me that a hallucinogenic experience allows one to look under the hood to reveal a truth that may be hidden in the subconscious mind. Even recreational use is healing in its own way. Psychedelic and entheogenic drugs are medicine.

Joshua and I dated while I was in law school, and we remained acquaintances. Hoping to strike up a new fling—because nope, I wasn't done trying to distract myself with men—I was disappointed when I realized that my attraction to him had waned. I couldn't tell if it was our time apart, his unkempt appearance, or my depression. I didn't flirt back but nonetheless, he offered me a bar of mushroom chocolate. I turned it over in my hands, noting that there was nothing to distinguish it from a regular bar of chocolate, except the wrapper looked like it was made with a home printer. With a wink and a cautionary smile, he didn't take any money for it. "Use it wisely," he told me.

One afternoon, I decided to eat most of the bar. Luke and Kristin would be gone all day, so I could do whatever I wanted. I told Kristin of my plan and while she was hesitant, she knew she couldn't stop me. I set up a chair in the sun in the fenced-in backyard of their small house and unrolled a yoga mat in case I wanted to stretch or roll around. Peppermint tea sat ready, as psychedelic mushrooms can sometimes induce nausea as they kick in. A neo-soul playlist curated especially for this purpose played as I set an intention for my psychedelic journey: "May I see truth."

The next few hours were a blur. I swayed to some of my old favorite songs until I couldn't stand the sound of music. Colors swirled and poignant memories came and went, as though I were watching a stylized reel of my life. At times agitated by the sunshine and feeling vulnerable outside, I'd go indoors. I sat in the living room on the oversized blue couch by the window. Kristin's English Mastiff dog, Chloe, kept my body company while my mind went on a journey. As I did on most days, I looked out the window longingly.

The difference was that this time I started to cry.

People outside were engaging with life with seeming ease, unaware of the undoing that was taking place within the tan house on Lowell Street. They were walking with their children and dogs, driving for errands, and picking up their mail. For months, I'd been unable to do any of these basic tasks, yet I thought I remembered a version of myself who could.

Where had she gone? It seemed impossible that I could have lost sight of her, but I couldn't find her.

I was an empty house.

No joy.

No hope.

No sense of self.

No value to the world.

No value to myself.

Nothing.

A pretense I'd been holding on to crumbled like a wall in the Acropolis. And with it a set of beliefs about myself and the world. That if I did the "right" thing—practice good law, be a good daughter, get married, use my gifts in service, do what I was "supposed" to do—I'd have a good life. I'd be perfect, happy, fulfilled, complete. Who was I in the absence of what I'd been told made a good life? Which parts of me developed to mask trauma, to feel worthy, to keep up my armor, to avoid being judged? Which parts of me were true?

The tears continued, and I wondered if I had finally broken. The floodgates wouldn't close despite my best efforts. After a few hours of being unable to stop, I called Kristin at work in desperation.

When she answered, I fought through the tears. "Something is wrong."

Her tone was urgent. "Are you okay?"

"No, no, no, no. I don't think so," I admitted, finally defeated.

I could hear her fighting to stay calm. "Okay. So what is wrong?"

She was met with silence and sobs. "Are you going to hurt yourself?" she asked. Suicide had crossed my mind, but only as an abstraction, never an act. I didn't want to die, necessarily. I just didn't want to feel like *this* anymore. The pain was too great.

"No, I won't." I was telling the truth.

"Promise me," she begged. "I'll be home in half an hour. Call your therapist and call me right back, okay? PROMISE ME!"

I called my therapist in L.A. She asked basic questions about how long ago I'd eaten the mushrooms and how I was currently feeling. "Broken," I told her. "I've finally broken." After listening to my situation and the flood of tears, she suggested an inpatient facility. "No," I said, vehemently and without hesitation. I thought about it. Then I said no again. *Hell* no. I had spent nine years in a prison of my own making at Legal Aid, and six months in the equivalent of solitary confinement at The Dungeon. There was not a chance in fuck I was going to a facility.

I would not commit myself to another place.

My therapist was familiar enough with my bullshit and self-justification to be unsurprised. She gently suggested I think about it and let it slide. Those *people need help, not me,* I thought.

And yet, I was one of "those people." I could not manage my life on my own. I could not go to work. I needed someone else to cook for me. I wouldn't eat without pressure. I needed someone to wash my clothes. I needed someone to pay my bills. I needed someone to hold me up. I needed someone to run my errands. I needed someone to dry my tears. I'd never felt so helpless and small. And I didn't know why I felt this way. Only that the feeling was overwhelming—and it blocked out everything good in my life and everything that felt good about being me.

Kristin flew through the door before I could finish my therapist call. Still in her work clothes, she sat with me on the couch for the next few hours while I finally shared with her how sick I was. When Luke came home, she took him aside and he disappeared again. That night, I cried everything left inside me as my sweet friend sat vigil, bearing witness to my little death. I had come undone.

For some, this psychedelic experience would have signaled "bad trip." For me, this was the most productive of them. Years of smiling, going through the motions, and pretending I was okay while depression ravaged my mind and body had taken their toll. I was powerless against it. I was finally able to see myself clearly and admit that I was desperately sick.

"We've got to talk about how we're going to get you healed," Kristin said to me gently the next day. "I know you well enough to know that you're not gonna go inpatient—right?"

I nodded emphatically.

"Okay, then, what about medication?"

"I don't want to take any drugs," I blurted.

Kristin's eyes widened and her mouth fell open. We both started laughing. I'd just eaten some psychedelic drugs the day before, and she *knew* me; I was no stranger to an altered state of consciousness. "You know what I mean!" I said, laughing. "Not *those* kinds."

I knew plenty of people who had gotten great results by using pharmaceutical medications to treat their depressions. My therapist had suggested them too many times to count. Yet I'd always been resistant to pills. I'm sure this was a stubborn remnant of my twisted idea of strength. It might also have stemmed from a healthy distrust of the Western medical system as a Black person. Aside from a daily thyroid replacement for multinodular thyroid disease and eight hundred milligrams of ibuprofen once a month to calm a uterus that seemed to choose violence to shed its lining, I didn't take anything else. Unsurprisingly, my end of life decisions for care and treatment request mostly holistic methods. We forward our values for living into our dying.

Further, I was unconvinced that my depression was due to a chemical imbalance. I'd already self-medicated and numbed myself with marijuana, wine, travel, and romance for too long. I was being called back to myself and it was time to heed the call. The mushrooms had shown me what I needed to see, and it was time to make a choice.

"So what's left?" Kristin pleaded.

I shrugged. No one else could tell me what I needed to do to heal. Or to live. Only I held the answers.

I decided to revisit my meditation practice, which had gone by the wayside. I needed to hear *me* again—my real thoughts, my actual reasons, my true desires, my underlying intentions, my truth. Since

I'd used my subconscious mind to see the problem, I wanted to try to use my conscious attention to heal it.

That's not a safe option for everybody, for sure. I wasn't even sure if it was the "right" course of action for me. But I felt compelled to try. I'd been a dedicated daily meditator for most of my adult life. But this time, when the going got tough, rather than double down on meditation, I stopped. It got too hard to be with myself—the good, the bad, the uncomfortable, and the hidden. Shadows, monsters, ghouls, and secrets. It can be a scary place, to sit still, particularly if you've gotten good at running, like I had. I needed to enter the liminal space.

Stillness isn't my forte. I walked before I was one year old, and I've been in motion ever since—fidgeting with my rings, hands, or clothes even when the rest of my body appears still. I can't handle any caffeine because it makes my insides itch. I use exercise to burn off the excess energy, but meditation helps me glimpse the stillness that my body can't seem to find otherwise. I get ants in my pants when I've been in one place too long, but my father has always reminded me that when I do not know where I am going, I should *be still*.

I didn't attempt real deal meditation until I had to survive law school. In college I'd picked up smoking both tobacco and weed, which allowed me to be with my breath, away from the noise and stimulation of parties. It was my first unintentional meditation. But in my early tries of mindfulness meditation, I'd sit, frustrated that I couldn't calm my mind long enough for anything to go still. Breathe in, breathe out—fidget, fidget, check time, move legs, touch hair. Fidget. Wonder what my crush in first grade was up to at that exact moment. *Where you at, Chad?* Fidget.

I almost gave up until I realized that my job wasn't to tame what meditators call "the monkey mind," but to observe it. To practice paying attention to where my mind chose to wonder, the ruts into which it fell. Meditation is a practice, after all. It is a practice of noticing the mind, but not quieting it. Of finding stillness in the liminal space, the space between two breaths.

We experience many liminal spaces while living. Stairways and elevators. Winter break. Airplanes and doorways. The interlude on Maxwell's *Urban Hang Suite*. The Brooklyn Bridge. Dusk. Dawn. Broken to breaking open. Birth, the quintessential transitional place. Through puberty, we sit between child and adult. When engaged, we are not single and not yet married. And as we lie actively dying, we are no longer of this world but not yet of whatever comes next, if anything at all. In culture, rites of passage mark our liminal spaces. In Western culture, few rituals exist to honor the liminality. Sitting vigil with the dying is one such ritual. Humans are notoriously uncomfortable with liminal spaces—which is why we sometimes need a guide to sit with us.

A young woman named Summer breezes into my life three months before her death. Knowing that it is soon approaching from a late-detected and terminal breast cancer, she wants to plan a home funeral to take the burden off her friends. She also wants to make sure she has the type of service *she* wants. At twenty-six years old and until recently estranged from her family, Summer's heard of death doulas and finds me courtesy of Instagram. Social media is a way for her to connect with other young cancer patients, feel connected to popular culture, and get support through her dying process.

By the time I meet Summer she has already begun to embrace her rapidly approaching death. "I'm supposed to be too young to die! But it's coming anyway!" she says. She is bracingly matter-of-fact, which is surprising given her age—fifteen years before doctors usually begin suggesting mammograms (and a good thirty years before people are "supposed" to get breast cancer). She'd ignored the lump in her breast her ex-boyfriend found a year earlier.

Her primary care doctor also didn't think much of it, given her age and unremarkable family history with the disease. When her lump was eventually biopsied, everything changed. The treatment plan was aggressive: chemo, radiation, and a double mastectomy. That worked for a short period, and Summer experienced the joys of remission. Then the cancer reemerged in her lymph nodes and quickly metastasized to the rest of her body. Her boyfriend left soon after.

I am in awe of how gracefully Summer shares this news with me, and I tell her so. At this admission, I wonder if I've put my big foot in my mouth. Without using the word, am I calling her "brave"—a dreaded word among the terminally ill? While it seems like a compliment, people living with serious illness don't have much of a choice about living with the disease. Illness is present. Cancer throws a shit avalanche at people and while there are choices in how to face it, merely living with illness doesn't make someone brave or heroic.

Many of my clients have told me that others encouraging their bravery and heroism disallowed them from expressing fear or anger. It encourages faking the funk by plastering on a smile. A sick person doesn't want to have to do that, nor should they have to. My own depression showed me that honesty can be a common victim of illness. I knew how easy it was to put on a brave smile, and how lonely it could be behind that smile.

Summer is no different. My rapport with her is easy and immediate. She wastes no time letting me know what's up. "While we're at it, please don't let anyone say I 'lost' my 'battle' with cancer, 'k?" She rolls her eyes and I groan theatrically.

The war analogy is so embedded in our language about disease. We say people "fight" cancer, or "lose" their lives, as though our bodies are not nature itself engaging in the regular ole cycle of birth, decay, and eventually death. When we use language of battle, we make winners and losers out of people we love when in reality, their bodies are either responding to treatment or not. Plenty of people who want to "win" against cancer still die. Did they not "fight" hard enough? Are they not "heroes"? Some feel empowered by the war metaphors and for them, they're useful. But it's most helpful to gain permission first before using such language to ensure that we are not alienating those who don't feel like fighters, valiant soldiers, or brave. Some are just sick and tired of being sick. They don't want to fight.

Even though she is dying, Summer is "winning" her bout with cancer, as far as I am concerned. She's still cheerleader-cute with a button nose and full lips, a blond, feathered, shoulder-length wig, and an attitude that recognizes since her time is soon up, she'd better be unapologetic about who she is. She continued horseback riding lessons when she felt well enough though treatment, and had her breasts reconstructed to the size she'd always wanted them to be: "34D-plus," as she calls them. "Too bad no one has played with these tattooed nipples," she says. When she offers to show them to me, I giggle and eagerly accept. She lifts her Rihanna T-shirt to show her newish, braless breasts. Her nipple tattoos look three-dimensional, with pinkish-brown areolas and little brown dots for the Montgomery glands that mask her scars. Even though I've only seen a few white women's boobs up close, I think these look pretty convincing.

"I love these super tits," she says while slowly shaking her shimmy and squeezing them. In another life where she isn't yet dying, the guests at Hooters would have loved her.

She gets sad when talking about not riding horses again. She vacillates between and holds joy and grief in a way that people decades her senior don't know is possible.

Her small home is cool in temperature, and two windows are open. It smells faintly sickly sweet—like caramel and medicine. Taking a look around, I wonder what she wants done with her possessions. She lives in a 425-square-foot studio garden guesthouse in the San Fernando Valley in Los Angeles with only a hot pot to cook her meals. Her kitchen counter is lined with dishes of various shapes and sizes and her shot glass collection. She's decorated the place with her hats and wooden blocks with calligraphy words written on them. No "live, laugh, love," but many other inspirational quotes. It feels like the first home of a young person—framed concert posters on the walls, twinkle lights behind the bed, a secondhand olive green couch acquired for free from craigslist. I feel a deep sadness knowing that her life will be over before she buys herself a new couch or switches out the posters for artwork.

I check myself again, but this time for the judgment and ageism that is rearing its head. Is Summer more deserving of my sadness because she hasn't yet marked adulthood in a way I deem meaningful? Summer's approaching death highlights one of my embedded harmful beliefs about people who die young. People often project their own fears about dying onto others. I am sad Summer hasn't had much experience as an adult, even though being an adult is not always fun. She left home and forged a life for herself when she was seventeen years old, finding a job, paying taxes, and snagging cost-efficient furniture that looks pretty good. At seventeen, I hadn't been kissed and only made $6.25 an hour at the movie theater. Perhaps she is more adult than I regard her as. I remind myself (again) to stop judging the life experiences of others.

Ageism is rampant in deathcare and in grief. It's well-meaning, but still not so nice. We tend to place greater emphasis on a person who dies young, ascribing greater misfortune to their death, while at the same time largely erasing the fact that young people die often too. When a young person dies, we call it a tragedy, since they "had their whole life ahead of them." What Summer has lived so far *is* her whole life. Denying this denies the absolute and sovereign timing of death.

"I don't care what happens to most of this stuff. I've already told my friends that they can take what they want, and the rest can be thrown away," she tells me. I ask about her sentimental possessions, but she hasn't amassed many recent ones. "My sister can have my

P!nk T-shirt, though." It's the first concert she went to. She'd left items from her youth in her childhood home when she fled after making allegations about her stepfather's sexual abuse. When her mother chose to side with her stepfather, Summer moved to L.A. from the Midwest, hoping to cash in on her looks in the film and TV industry. But she struggled to find an agent or work beyond being cast as an extra, and she decided to stop communicating with her family. As the end of her life approaches, Summer changes her mind and reconnects with her mom, Betsy, and younger sister, Georgia. Upon hearing that Summer's cancer will end her life, they come to L.A. to be Summer's caregivers and plan to stay until she dies. On this day I'm visiting, Betsy and Georgia have stepped out to give Summer and me some time to ourselves. I suspect they also aren't ready for the frank conversation we are about to have about Summer's funeral. She wants an alternative one—a home funeral.

Summer has decided that she wants to be laid out at home for a few hours after she dies. She's seen a video about home funerals and since her friend group in L.A. got much smaller through her treatment, she wants those closest to her to have some time with her body before she is cremated. After relying heavily on these friends through her treatment, she doesn't want to start another crowd-sourcing campaign to pay for anything else. Her ashes are to be sent home with her mom. Imagining her ideal deathbed, Summer focuses on orange roses, her favorite flower. With this detail we envision a deathbed where the flowers are placed on her bed and body and decorate her apartment. The Lumineers song "Don't Wanna Go" will play as her few loved ones gather.

She plays it for me. Listening to the lyrics, tears come to my eyes. Despite the fact that I have been with many clients, I always feel strong emotion in the presence of someone whose life will end soon. It doesn't make me any less professional. It just makes me human.

Through my work, I've learned to love people who are leaving. It's a hazard of the job. Inevitably, they die. And while I know it's coming because it's the precise reason why we are working together, it doesn't make it any easier. In some ways, it's harder. I know all of their fears of death, their worries for their families, concerns about the messes they might leave. And I know that they journey directly into it anyway. There is no choice. It makes me love them more.

Summer is emotional too. She doesn't want to die, but she knows her time is near. She is ill. In the months that we've been working together, her appearance has changed. Hollowed cheeks. Gray pallor. Slow movements. Slurred words. Blue veins visible under her skin, especially over her new breasts. Her life light is fading. And she is clear about how she wants that light to go out.

After making plans for her body to be removed after her death by a company that will directly cremate her, and discussing that her implants will have to be removed before the cremation, we talk a little about religion. Like me, Summer was raised an evangelical Christian. And also like me, she never really vibed with the idea of heaven and hell. She rejected Christianity after she left home and hasn't looked back. Until now.

"What if I'm wrong?" she asks, drawing out her syllables.

"Right? Like what if we should have gone to church every Sunday?" I respond playfully.

"Or if we shouldn't fucking curse!"

"Well, you're about to find the fuck out! Let me know, okay?"

We laugh about it, but I keep the conversation about religion going since it seems to be on her heart. The deathbed is the most important time for what's most pressing on our hearts to take center stage. Soon there will be no more time to talk about our heart's burdens. By the end of our session, Summer has chosen which parts of Christianity she wants to keep and has decided that she would like to get baptized. Just in case. Although she doesn't believe that she will go to hell for rejecting Christianity and living secularly, she still harbors some doubt. Better safe than burn in eternal damnation.

I celebrate her choice just as I would if she were Muslim, Buddhist, Hindu, or a whirling dervish.

The way I doula places secularity at its core. The needs of clients from differing religions are pretty universal. This allows me to stay secular in my approach to help them prepare for dying. We generally all die the same, except for what we believe comes after. I can support clients to get clear on what they believe without muddying the space with what I believe. Also what I believe changes, shifts, and redefines through every death I attend and day I live, so it's a crapshoot on any given day.

I chat this over with the hospice chaplain, who is tickled at Summer's eleventh-hour conversion. So am I. And so is her mother, who's been begging Summer to come back to church since she left home. She is finally getting her wish—her baby will go to heaven, according to her beliefs. I can tell how much this means to her. My parents would probably be ecstatic too. Pastor Joe performs the baptismal rites, sprinkles some water on her head, and thanks God for forgiveness for Summer's sins. When he leaves she says, "Some of those sins were really fun to make. Is it okay that I'm not sorry for them?" Her levity is balm for my spirit, and I tell her that I'll ask Pastor Joe on her behalf (and a little on my behalf too).

Since Summer's time to die seems to be approaching, I visit her again the next afternoon. Walking through the patio door into her room, I can tell something is different. Summer is sitting in bed and pulling at her sheets, feebly trying to uncover her feet and lift herself up. Even though she only weighs about as much as my left leg, she isn't able to get herself up, as disease has withered her muscle tone. Repeatedly, she mumbles that she needs her suitcase and that she wants to leave. She's frustrated, a marked departure from our visits before. There is a quality to her behavior I've seen in clients close to death. I offer to help uncover her feet but it doesn't help.

Recognizing her behavior as terminal agitation, I ask where she wants to go in case I am wrong. Summer mutters mostly to herself but in response to my question, "Somewhere. I dunno. Somewhere else. Anywhere but here. I want to go. Help me." But there is nowhere to go. Active dying is near. Terminal agitation (sometimes called terminal restlessness or hyperactive delirium) is the anxiety, agitation, and confusion that is present at the end of life but more marked than the mood swings that accompany dying. The dying person may seem angry, distressed, impatient, restless, and unable to relax. The metabolic and physiological changes one undergoes while the body's systems shut down may be one of the causes, but no one really knows. I wonder if it is a last-ditch effort to try to escape death. Antianxiety medications can relieve the symptoms and are often prescribed by hospice teams when available.

Betsy tells me that Summer has recently been given pain medication, so we can rule uncontrolled pain out as a cause of her distress. Georgia is upset that her sister is being curt with her. I explain to Georgia that Summer's behavior is likely because of her dying process. I'm not sure how much it helps. The nurse will soon be on her way to check for other causes of distress. Until the nurse arrives, I sit with Betsy, Summer, and Georgia and try to calm her using the playlist she'd made that she'd told me would help her through emotional distress. Summer's playlist sounds like what you'd hear in a yoga nidra class. Music choices are part of a standard conversation I have early in my end of life planning work with clients: together we make a list of simple comforts, rituals, nurturing words, music, poetry, and texts or religious verses to help them through the emotional distress of dying.

When the nurse arrives, he confirms Summer's symptoms. She is not reporting any pain. The nurse asks me to prepare Betsy and Georgia for what is coming; we've gotten close, and he trusts me to deliver this news. I explain to them what to expect in the coming days and make myself available for whatever they might need for the night ahead. They've been understandably upset by Summer's misery but are grateful to hear that relief would soon be coming, even if that relief is death. After Summer falls into a deep sleep, I head home for some rest, knowing the days ahead will be transformative. Each death is.

I only sleep with the ringer on when a client is actively dying. Sleep quality is poor anyway knowing that someone I've come to care for is making their departure. This night is no different. Normally, I leave it up to the family as to whether they'd like me to be there close to the moment of death. Some want me there with them, and others just want to know that someone cares. Others need questions answered, and others call after the death has occurred. It's all okay with me, as long as they feel supported. Summer herself has requested that I be there for her death and Betsy eagerly agrees. I otherwise trust my clients in their innate ability to die.

Disoriented, I wake up at 7 A.M. to the shrill ringing phone and make a mental note to change it to something that sounds less like military trucks signaling that war has arrived in my town. Summer's breathing has changed significantly, and Betsy hasn't slept a wink, intently focused on her inhales and exhales. They are jagged and slowing down over the last hour. Death won't be long. Quickly splashing cold water on my face, I brush my teeth, grab a protein bar, and head off to sit vigil with Summer in her liminal space.

When entering a room where dying is imminent, I pause before walking in, reminding myself to treat each death like it's my first. In ritual, I touch the doorframe in a reminder that I am crossing a threshold. Whoever I meet on the other side will change me. The Alua who enters will not be the Alua who leaves. Death changes everyone. Silently, I repeat the mantra I've adopted for myself for this work: *May I speak truth. May I speak love. May I be my highest blessing.*

Like active labor, active dying is an equally juicy liminal space, deserving of total sacredness and honor. After all, dying is the space between here and there (wherever there is). In most natural deaths, there are a few recognizable signs that death is near. In the days and hours before death, the dying individual begins to disengage with people in their lives and their attention turns inward. Kidney function slows, reducing and darkening urine output. Blood pressure drops, as does body temperature. The extremities are cool to the touch and the skin turns blotchy, which is called mottling. This is also evident in darker-skinned people. In this liminal space, the eyelids fall slightly open, but the individual no longer responds to stimulus appearing in front of the eyes. The mouth then falls open and breathing patterns become irregular. Life hangs on a single breath.

As I enter the room, I can feel the shift in energy. A stillness has started descending, which will blanket the room when Summer leaves it. I center myself for what is to come, knowing fully that there is nothing to do but hold space for and bear witness to this inexplicable event. I am so lucky to get to stand in the doorway to existence, walk in, and walk out, transformed by the power of life and death.

Crossing the threshold, I set my death doula bag of tricks by the door. The cute Moroccan camel-leather duffel bag holds a few items for ritual: books of poetry, a singing bowl, blank paper, candles, essential oils, incense, matches, Agua Florida, a pouch of dirt, and a pouch of tea leaves; and items the family can use in natural death-care: cotton balls, underpads, washcloths, hair ties, tissues, lotion, Castile soap, a hairbrush, and a small bowl for washing. My doula bag also holds a bottle of water, an apple, Cheez-Its, a phone charger, and whatever juicy novel I might be reading at the time. Gotta stay hydrated and balanced. There are also various fabrics to dress up a space, just in case.

Betsy holds a tissue worn to fluffy strings of cotton in one hand and her daughter's left hand in the other. Her eyes are bloodshot and her hair is disheveled. One look at Summer confirms that she is actively dying. Her weakened and irregular pulse reinforces it. In a whisper, I tell her I will kiss her, before I place one on her forehead and notice that her button nose has started to turn bluish at the tip. This is cyanosis—another sign of active dying. Her brown eyes are slightly open but not responsive to any stimulus. Her mouth lies slack and her breathing has turned mechanical, slowing to about seven to ten breaths a minute. The body is doing its job to shut itself down. I grab the orange roses from outside that Summer loves and put them on the nightstand. Then, per her request, I put one in her hand. I kiss her again and whisper again that she is doing it right.

For the next three hours, I alternate between rubbing Betsy's back, singing songs, hugging Georgia and reminding her to breathe, holding Summer's hand and counting her breaths. They slow to six breaths a minute then speed up. This is likely a breathing pattern called Cheyne-Stokes breaths. The space between her inhales and exhales is short and sharp, yet a seeming eternity passes between each. Together, we hang in this liminal space with Summer, also holding our breaths with her until she does not inhale again.

Summer has died. And then, the sacred stillness envelopes and holds us all. It is ripe with wonder of life and the awe of death. Betsy and Georgia tearfully and reverently wash her body with my instruction, rubbing a washcloth dipped in lavender oil–scented water over her face, arms, torso, and legs.

Together we change her into a crocheted white gown she'd chosen prior to her death. We spread orange roses around her. The friends she'd asked me to call come to her house, dressed in white. She'd also wanted them to wear the hats she'd collected, so they each put one on—a motley assortment of trucker hats, cowboy hats, bowlers, and fedoras. One by one, they say their goodbyes as the others mill about, nibbling on snacks and consoling each other. She's also asked that they each have a shot and take a glass with them. I take a shot but leave the glass for someone else.

After an hour or so Pastor Joe comes and leads us in a Christian funeral, including a short sermon. Understanding the significance of a recently converted and dead Christian, he weaves it into the service and we sing secular songs of Summer's choosing. When it is over, we hold hands around her body until the crematory comes to take her body away while the Lumineers' song plays.

The grief at Summer's death looks just like it does when an elderly person dies. Looking around, I see the same grief—bowed heads, murmured voices, quiet tears—that I would have at an elderly grandparent's funeral. Yet culturally we would expect the grief to be greater because Summer was young. Ageism in death also rears its head when expressing condolences. In grief, ageism sounds like "She lived a long, full life" or " You got sixty-five good years with her" when talking about the deaths of older people, even if those years were shit. When we say that someone who died lived a "long, full life," we end up unintentionally minimizing the grief experience for the person who is grieving the death of an elderly person. Can they still not be sad, even if Grandma was old? Who can say if someone died too soon? Or if they experienced everything they wanted to? Maybe Grandma wanted to fall in love one last time and her prospects were cut short by only living ninety-seven years. It hurts no matter what.

Summer was young at the time of her death, and her body was no longer responding to treatment. But she was healing. There is healing available in death even though we often think of health as the antithesis of death. The word *healing* often indicates that something can change and improve for the better, yet we know that a person cannot be "cured" from death. The best we can do is bring comfort to the dying process and support in healing emotional and spiritual wounds. Sometimes "healing" is leaving a sick body.

In her dying, Summer healed her relationship with her body. This was evident in her chosen metaphor—she was in a "dance" with cancer and did not make her illness the villain—and in her pride in showing off her freshly tattooed nipples. She healed her relationship with her family and healed her relationship with religion through her death. She reconciled the life she'd had with the one she'd wanted. Summer had the good death that many dream of, even if many might believe she "should" have had a longer life. But because she died when she did, her life was complete after all.

Chapter 16

Cuba Te Espera

If there was one question I could ask the Creator/La Luna/Prince/ the Orishas/the magical love force that knows all, I'd simply ask: Why?

Why the heartache? Why depression? Why mosquitos? Why all the pain, the insecurity, the uncertainty, and most of all, why life itself? Why death?

The "why" of life is ever so potent when greeting death. The urge to know the answer is strong, and our emotional need for it can feel so urgent, so overwhelming. Sometimes, a client straight *demands* to know the answer, looking to me as if I'll reveal all of life's great mysteries for a fee. I have compassion for them. It is all I can do, in those cases, to help them gaze into that unknown, and to hold them in their fear and doubt about whether their lives were good enough. I know that fear well, myself.

When I meet Leslie, she greets me, breathless, on the front steps to her humble apartment. At sixty-seven years old, she's been hooked up to an oxygen machine that has been her constant companion for months. She is in the late stages of a lung disease that has hardened her airways and the few steps from the armchair to open the front door make her lose her breath.

Leslie's apartment is decorated with various knickknacks—porcelain owls, framed decorative spoons, Russian dolls, pictures of her only daughter, Kathleen. Kathleen has called me to support her mother, who is struggling to come to terms with the disease that will end her life. I help Leslie get back to the armchair, which is in her main living area, facing the door and window. In the twelve steps between the front door and the chair, we stop twice.

She lowers herself into the chair and reaches for the side table, which has everything she needs over the course of the day to steady herself. Remote control. Medications. A book of daily Christian devotions. Cell phone and landline. Tissues. A bag of almonds. Her daughter's picture. The dirty plate, with remnants of breakfast. A notebook and a pen, which she gathers from the table.

We exchange pleasantries, and then Leslie cuts bracingly to the point: "What does dying feel like?"

It's her first question. In all the years I've done this, I have never been asked this question so directly. I'm floored. "Oh. Well, I don't know," I stammer. "But since I have been around a few people who are dying, I can tell you what they have shared about their experiences while they could still communicate. Would that be helpful?"

"Mmm, not quite," Leslie responds. "I really want to know what the moment of death actually feels like."

I am at a loss. "I don't know. I haven't done it yet, so I can't speak from experience."

She cocks her head to the side and looks at me quizzically. "Okay, then let's move on." Leslie draws a line on the page, presumably through the question she just asked, and scans her questions again. "What happens after we die?"

I feel a smidge of relief—not because I know the answer, of course, but because I'm asked this question constantly. Most of us have some beliefs about what happens after we die, but people who are at the end of their lives are particularly confronted with it. Beliefs are often like a murky lake for those on the precipice about to jump in. There will soon be evidence about what lies at the bottom. The best I can do is help people get clear about what they think happens. I've noticed that even the most religious among us quietly begin to second-guess their beliefs when they know they will soon find out the answer.

"I don't know that answer either," I tell Leslie, "since I'm still here with the living."

As a rule, I don't much discuss my viewpoint about an afterlife with my clients. It's private. Plus, I want to be an unstreaked mirror for the dying, as they work through their own ideas. It is *their* death. I get to have mine later. In a classic doula move, I turn the question back to Leslie. "What do *you* believe happens when we die?"

"I don't think it matters what I believe since I want to know what actually happens," she answers. "Can you help me with that?" She takes another pained breath as the oxygen machine next to her whirs softly.

"I can't tell you for sure since no one who has been all the way there has ever been back to tell us," I say. I tell her that it might be more helpful to talk about what she's come to believe, because we pick up bits and pieces from religion, science, culture, movies, our fears, etc. But Leslie cuts me off. "I don't want to play the guessing game," she insists. "I want to know. Are you telling me that you don't have the answer?"

Fearing I am failing her but seeing no way through, I nod. "You're right. I don't know. I can't know for sure until I die."

"Okay." Returning to her notebook and forcefully drawing another line on the page, crossing out the question, Leslie continues. "Is dying painful?"

Finally, a question I can answer with some clarity. "From what I understand, dying itself isn't painful. The pain that people experience at the end of life is typically a function of the disease process, and not from dying itself. Your hospice team will be well equipped to give you pain medication so that you are not uncomfortable while you die."

"So you're saying that I won't be in pain?"

"I'm saying that any pain you experience from your disease should be well controlled by your doctors. We can talk to your doctors about your concerns and make a plan to address them. Does that ease your mind a bit?"

"Kinda. I want to know if it will hurt."

"It shouldn't."

Leslie takes a few more breaths and stares at her notebook blankly. I can't tell if she just needs a moment to gather her thoughts or if she is growing impatient with me. She flips the page and drags her pen down it, lingering for a moment halfway down the page.

"When I lose consciousness, how much longer will I have before I am dead?"

Shit. I am starting to feel useless. "It varies from one person to the next. Some people die really quickly after they close their eyes for the final time, and others hang out in the in-between space for days. There is no way to know for sure what your process will be."

Leslie exhales sharply. It could be her disease, although it sure sounds a lot like impatience. "Can I communicate with my daughter after I die?"

Here is another bit I can work with. I can talk with Leslie about the parts of consciousness she believes exist after we die. We can talk about the little inside jokes she shares with her daughter. We can explore the ways in which Kathleen will feel close to her mother after her death when she hears those key words or images. I can share stories I've heard about hummingbirds and butterflies that refused to leave the sides of those who are grieving. But I am losing faith that any of this would serve as an adequate answer to Leslie's questions.

The real work we are doing together emerges. Leslie is grappling with the great unknowns of death and the surrender it requires. For most of her questions, there is simply no adequate answer. I wonder if, deep down, she knows this. Perhaps a spiritual advisor would have been better for her, and I suggest that she also ask these questions of the chaplain on the hospice team. Maybe I could have offered pithy platitudes or told her whatever I imagined she wanted to hear. Sometimes I wonder if it is the more compassionate thing to do. But the true answer to most of the questions about death is "I don't know."

I ask Leslie whether she'd felt any communication with the people in her life who had already died. She tells me her dead aunt's favorite decorative spoon is the only one that falls off the wall from time to time, and that she loves that her aunt is quietly telling her that she is still there. She softens toward me a bit as she flips through her notebook again. After a thick uncomfortable silence, she asks tentatively, "How much time do I have left?"

My heart breaks. I smile a soft smile and bravely hold her gaze. I say nothing.

"Let me guess," she says. "You don't know." She exhales. I hold my breath.

Finally Leslie shuts her notebook with some force. I am right that she has grown impatient. "So what *do* you know?"

"Not much, clearly!"

We chuckle uncomfortably.

"So what are you here for?" Leslie asks with a sigh.

I explain my role as a companion and offer to support her in the tasks she can control. I assure Leslie that she is asking all of the right questions and doing all of the hard work. Reminding her that the questions she asks are ones that no earthly person can answer, I encourage her to stay immersed in the questions. Some do not require an answer. Some have no answer at all. This is the hard part of dying. It is also the hard part of living. How can we stay present with today not knowing if there is a tomorrow?

In elementary school we are taught that you can gather enough information to aid in problem-solving if you answer five basic *W* questions: who, what, when, where, why. However, it's not remotely helpful when thinking about death. When applying the five *W* formula from our elementary school education, it is without use.

Who dies? Everyone. No one in the history of time has escaped death.

What is death? Science and experience tell us that death is the cessation of all critical bodily functions and activities necessary to sustain life.

When do we die? Unless a person chooses the date and time of their death, it will remain unknown until that very last breath.

Where do we die? See "when," above.

Why do we die? Major religions, philosophers, and people on mind-altering substances have grappled with this question forever. And no one seems to have an answer good enough to appease us.

No wonder death makes us so uncomfortable. We can't gather much information about it, and gathering information is what makes us feel safe. Thinking about death drives us directly into the discomfort of "I don't know." In my work supporting people through dying, I meet many who cling to what they think they can control, to avoid surrendering to life's biggest "I don't know."

Getting comfortable with the "I don't know"s in death work has humbled me. No certainty exists in the practice of death companioning. At times it leaves me feeling powerless to help my clients. I can't take away their discomfort over the uncertainty, nor can I provide information to make it more comfortable. I can't fix their fear. The best I can do is be there with them as they try to create answers for themselves, while practicing surrendering into the unknown. There are things we can control, such as handling our affairs and saying our "I love you"s and "you hurt me"s. But the big questions will always remain unanswered.

Getting comfortable with the "I don't know"s in life has also humbled me. Life is an "I don't know." We don't know what will happen in the next minute. When we are present to this, we feel piddly, pathetic, and powerless. So we busy ourselves, staving off the existential dread with chores, tasks, addiction, work, sex, and anything else we can do to avoid our discomfort.

When we open ourselves up to the discomfort of not knowing, that's where all the juice lies. When we think we know, we are not pliable. We are stagnant and stuck. Opening ourselves up to the discomfort of not knowing means opening ourselves up to the magic of what may be—the place of pure boundless potential where anything is possible. It allows the humans we meet along the way to guide us back to ourselves and our individual truth. Life unfurls before us. This is the only knowing available. The unknown is precisely what makes us human. I rely on this truth with every client.

Leslie dies less than a year after our initial meeting. In the time between our first meeting and her death, I come to her home and sit with her several more times. Her big questions remain, but rather than looking to me for answers, she's getting comfortable with not knowing and listening to her own truth—the only one that matters. My job both as a death doula and a human is merely to witness her in the discomfort and her vulnerability of not knowing what's to come, and to hold her there until she finds out the truth for herself.

In my favorite movies, the main character always experiences a blinding revelation: Celie finds her power and curses Mister in *The Color Purple*, and Cher Horowitz realizes she's in love with her stepbrother, Josh, in *Clueless*. There are big fireworks and a fountain erupts as it dawns on her.

In real life, the truth of who we are and what we want doesn't often reveal itself in one climactic moment. The path toward personal truth is slower, maddening, excruciating, and piecemeal. Life leaves us bread crumbs to follow. It is up to us to follow these bread crumbs down the path, one by one. They can lead us somewhere that finally feels like home. At the end, we might have an "I love Josh!" moment ourselves.

I was one of Leslie's bread crumbs.

Elián González, of all people, was one of mine.

After a few frustrating weeks trying to settle into my meditation practice at Kristin's, where time moved like molasses and my mind wouldn't stop wandering, my practice started to stick. As if on well-worn train tracks, my mind constantly wandered back to my disease and whether I would get healthy again. I wondered how I'd gotten here and about the choices I'd made. I wondered about my mistakes and people I'd hurt. I wondered about my ex-boyfriends and how they put up with my flighty, noncommittal nature. I wondered if my family would be heartbroken about how much I'd been hurting.

During one morning meditation, my mind wandered to Elián. A Cuban citizen, he emigrated to the United States in an inner tube with his mother. She drowned along the way and Elián, who was six years old at the time, was thrown into an international custody battle between his relatives in the US and his father in Cuba. Elián must have also been in the deepest grief. His name dominated the news; you couldn't enter a gas station without hearing about him.

In June 2000, a US court of appeals ruled that Elián had to be returned to Cuba and he was forcefully removed from the home of his paternal relatives. The front page of every newspaper showed the image of a scared little boy with Border Patrol guns pointed at him and his uncle, hiding in a closet. I was horrified at the force used to retrieve a child, and the image haunted me for months.

Twelve years later in meditation, Elián's face resurfaced in my mind and I couldn't shake him.

After that, I was eager to find out what had happened to Elián. I learned that he had become a member of the Cuban army, which led me down a rabbit hole. I read about the United States embargo, the Cuban missile crisis, the Cold War, and the history of Cuba's leadership. I looked at Cuba's geography and culture. I was reminded that one of my favorite bands, the Buena Vista Social Club, was from Cuba.

I was intrigued in that way that felt familiar to me. I was also wary of my own tendencies: In one of the toughest moments of my life, was I seeking out another distraction? Why was I so curious about him?

Unclear on the answers, I dragged myself away from the computer and ate the baby carrots and hummus Kristin had left for me on the counter that morning. Then I headed to the library on Luke's red Schwinn ten-speed, pumping my legs against the pedals, wind in my hair. I was returning a book called *Dying to Be Me*. It's the memoir of a doctor, Anita Moorjani, whose organs failed after a dance (not a battle) with cancer. She details her near-death experience and comes to acknowledge the root of her disease, thereby healing herself. The book had jumped off the shelf when I was at the library a few days earlier. I was inspired and wondered if I could find the root of my disease and heal myself.

When I got to the library, there were a few people milling about with petitions I was not in the mood to sign. Despite the bike ride and listening to the Buena Vista Social Club all morning during my Cuba/Elián deep dive, I was grouchy and irritated. I'd been that way for months—depression's fault. But the library was one of the few places that lifted my spirits. I was looking forward to getting inside. Reading books still provided a reliable ticket outside myself. I returned the Moorjani book and grabbed a few more: *The Witch of Portobello* by Paulo Coelho, *My Sister's Keeper* by Jodi Picoult, and *Quantum Healing* by Deepak Chopra.

Outside the library, a lanky young man holding a clipboard tried to catch my eye. "Excuse me, miss!" He raised his voice while he moved toward me.

I looked to the ground and kept walking. *Isn't this universal language for* leave me alone? Evidently, he didn't speak it.

"Hi, do you have a minute for the environment?"

"No, I'm really busy," I lied, knowing damn well I didn't have any place else to be for months. The man followed me.

"It will only take a minute. Have you ever heard of Greenpeace?"

Turns out it didn't matter, because he was gonna tell me anyway. As the fellow extolled the virtues of the environmental organization, his squeaky voice all out of proportion to his tall, sinewy frame, I felt my heart soften. His passion for his work made me slow my pace. After talking with me about the dangers of climate change and its effects on the rainforest, he made the pitch: "So would you consider donating?"

I told him I was on a fixed budget and asked if there was something I could sign instead. He kept pushing, and I started to get impatient. I had a whole lot of nothing to get back to! Finally getting the picture that he would get no money from me, the man offered me a Greenpeace pamphlet as a parting gift. He reached into an old, dark blue leather messenger bag to retrieve it. It had cracks on the single strap and a few frayed strings hanging off it. Across the front, emblazoned in red, were the Spanish words *Cuba te espera*.

I motioned impatiently toward his bag. "What does that mean?" I knew the answer with my rudimentary Spanish, but I still looked outside myself for an answer.

The young man looked confused. "You mean this?" he asked, pointing to the slogan. "It means 'Cuba is waiting.'"

I caught my breath. My eyes narrowed. Juicebumps.

Apparently, *Cuba te espera* was an advertising slogan from the days when Cuba was widely open to U.S. tourists. Nowadays, there is no getting there for Americans (at least not officially) unless there is a legitimate learning purpose. The guidelines seemed strict, and only to be violated by the adventurous. Or the foolish. Or the desperate. I was all three.

"Have you been to Cuba?" I ask, my curiosity piquing by the second.

No, he answered, but a few friends of his had. "You've got to go through Mexico or one of the Caribbean islands so you can do whatever you want there," he told me. "You also have to tell them not to stamp your passport when you get there because if you get caught, there could be a hefty fine for not following the rules."

I nodded slowly, leaning toward him, hanging on to his every word. "I was researching Cuba this morning," I told him tentatively. I went on to mention Elián González and some of his life updates I'd just read about.

This guy was way too young to remember Elián. He squinted at me, politely uncomprehending.

I nodded at his bag. "You think this is a sign?"

Shielding my eyes with one hand from the sun, I waited for a response from this clipboard-toting kid. I was desperate and would have accepted anything, from anyone, as confirmation that Cuba was a good idea. I saw everything as a clue about how to get out of depression.

The young man shrugged, while I tried to ignore the champagne bubbles forming in my blood. "Might be," he offered.

That was enough for me.

I raced home on the Schwinn with my backpack full, my heart near bursting from exertion. It was the fastest I'd moved in months. Throwing my backpack on Paco, my trusty sleeping pad, I hurried back to the desk I'd left only an hour earlier. The search page I'd left open about the Cuban missile crisis was still open.

A few hours later, I'd found a route through Cancún and a tourism company that would help me complete official documents to enter the country legally, using the educational purpose loophole. The tour was strict as to not violate the U.S. travel restrictions—but after the first three days, I was going to go AWOL and travel on my own. I just needed the tour company to get into the country and to get my treasured passport stamp legally.

The plan was coming together seamlessly—except for the fact that I was clinically depressed, hadn't cooked myself a meal in six months, and relied on Kristin for my most basic needs. How was I going to navigate international travel by myself? I didn't know but I didn't care. I was still doing stupid shit. But Cuba was waiting.

Before Kristin got home from work and could talk me out of it,

I'd booked a flight to Cancún for two weeks from that date. I figured that would be enough time to regain some basic life skills, learn a little Spanish, and convince my family and friends that I would be fine traveling alone. Right?

All the legal training in the world couldn't have prepared me for the fight everyone put up when I told them I was going to Cuba by myself. I protested that I'd been traveling alone internationally for fifteen years. Kristin reminded me of the day I cried for hours over my missing shoe. My therapist asked how I'd be able to get in touch with her. My mom—always nervous about my international travels anyway—could barely disguise the worry in her voice. I could see her furrowed eyebrows and rounded shoulders over the phone: "Oh, okay," she said, her telltale response to one of my cockamamie ideas.

My sisters tried to convince me to go the next year.

My dad reminded me that Cuba has terrible international relations with the U.S.

They were all correct. It was a terrible idea. And I was listening to the exact same voices that had propelled me all around the world in search of myself only to wind up with nothing. After all, I'd spent the last decade leaping into escape pod after escape pod whenever I hit a rough patch. How could I be sure that Elián and his heartrending story wasn't an excuse I was beginning to concoct, to sow chaos and run from my life, when what I needed was to stay still, confront it, and find some peace?

I'd found an inkling of peace in my meditation practice, but the deeply ingrained impulses that send us running away from ourselves run far deeper than inklings. Sometimes these impulses crash us directly back into ourselves and force us to confront something we've always known but fear to acknowledge.

All I knew then was that I felt a hint of a tingle in my blood for the first time in—I couldn't remember how long. Everything in my life, at that moment, was a big NO. Cuba felt like a thundering YES. I had to go, even as I fought with myself about it. Each night I tossed and turned, nightmares of being lost in the country with no one to rescue me. It was a possibility. Would I fall back into old habits and patterns? I'd tried this "travel cure" before and it never worked. What was that old line about the definition of insanity? What made me sure this time something would be different?

But the little bit of light I had inside my body—the tingle that whispered "Cuba is waiting"—was louder than my fear. I told my parents I'd email them daily, and they would share the info with my sisters. I planned a lengthy check-in with my therapist once a week. I promised to continue my meditation practice. I gave myself permission to not have the answers. To take my time. To fuck it up. To tell myself the truth about how I was feeling. And to forgive myself regularly. To hold myself with all the tenderness of a baby bird. I felt like one. Fragile. A walking nerve ending.

Kristin's home had been a womb. For six weeks, I'd let myself be needy. I'd let Kristin see all of my broken parts and let her help me put them back together. Now, I was walking back into the world, whether I was ready or not.

At the airport, finally walking away from her into the terminal, I shivered. I worried I wouldn't remember to eat. I stood at the terminal, looking at the "Cancún" sign. Was I the same me, going around in the same sad circles, or was something . . . different? If so, was it me or the situation that had changed? I couldn't be sure.

After all, here I was again, running again. Was I succumbing to boredom and restlessness once more? I had come to think of my restlessness as my Achilles' heel—the fatal flaw guaranteed to keep me unhappy. Restlessness was that voice screaming at me to put down the paperwork, to break up with the partner, to book tickets to dubious locales. It was the voice that kept me unfocused in school, unreliable at work, flighty in love. I had been locked in a mortal battle with that voice for so long and had suffered so much.

And yet.

Maybe the voice hadn't caused my suffering. Maybe, instead, my suffering had come from my refusal to heed it. Maybe I was forever fidgeting because I was fighting against the urgent message it was sending me. Maybe what I needed, finally, was to wake up to that voice inside of me, and acknowledge, finally and fully, what it was trying to tell me:

ONE DAY YOU ARE GOING TO DIE.

It is the simplest truth of them all, and yet it is the one we fight the hardest.

We push it away. We procrastinate. Death is something that happens to *other* people, or else to us in a future so distant it's the same thing as "never." We prioritize all the things that matter the least at the expense of those that matter most.

People wait entire lifetimes to see the Great Wall of China until they are too sick to travel, and save the bottle of Veuve Clicquot till they can't drink anymore.

We wait till tomorrow to make that important phone call, until Friday to wear the purple lipstick, or for the summer to start working on the clubhouse for the kids. Before we know it, we have an illness, then a diagnosis, then we are knocking at death's door.

Life is now. It's right here. This is it.

The past is just a series of memories coded in the hippocampus. Tomorrow, forever a day away, is a myth and an illusion of our brain's insistence on linear time. *This* moment is the only one that exists. In the very next moment, you could also be gone, a memory in someone else's hippocampus.

As it turns out, having a personality like mine—passionate, sensitive, creative, curious, quirky—has made me uniquely awake to this truth. As a lawyer, my impatience for bureaucracy and focus on ultimate truths and compassion had me crawling out of my skin. In death work, this focus helps me be present with my clients and to help them be present with themselves. Firmly rooted in my body. My habit of forever seeking without any promise of finding helps me guide clients through the terror of the unknown. If there was an answer to the eternal *why*, I wouldn't want it. This way, I can keep savoring the delicious mystery of every facet of existence. Who I am is not a defect. Who I am is a gift.

So yes, I was running away from something as I waited for my flight to Cuba. But I was also running *toward* something. I didn't know why or who it was yet, but I knew she was there somewhere. I found her in Cuba on a Viazul bus, in the electrifying company of a German woman traveling the world to see what she could see, before uterine cancer might end her life. I found her by imagining myself on my deathbed for the first time. And with my death as my guide, I will find her over and over again, continuing to follow my curiosities, my truth, and my bliss until—at last—I die too.

Every single person I've had the honor of accompanying toward their death has left me with an invaluable lesson about life, showing me the myriad ways you can choose to live it—and die. They all live inside of me, and their lessons do too.

But when it comes to following your truth fearlessly, naysayers be damned, there are few who moved me as much as Ms. Bobbie.

I meet Ms. Bobbie a few years after I start my death work practice. Her daughter has asked me to sit with her once a week on the days she and her sister can't be there as a companion. In a short time it becomes clear that my work with Ms. Bobbie is to do a long-life review, strolling down memory lane and creating some context to her life. I glean this from the stories Ms. Bobbie tells and retells as she keeps her focus on the past and the life she created in an attempt to wind it down. Nothing remains undone in her life, and there are no tasks left to complete.

Born in 1923, Ms. Bobbie has just turned ninety-four years old and is confined to a bed in an eldercare facility in Los Angeles after she'd lost the ability to live by herself. Her bed is the first of three, separated by curtains in a dim room, farthest from the old box television bolted to the top right corner. Parkinson's disease has shriveled her hands, and her legs can no longer hold her body's weight. Yet her spirit is full, and Ms. Bobbie is enthusiastic for company. "Baby, look at you! You came to see me looking goooood!" she says with twinkling eyes every time I walk in the door, so I make sure to dress up for her and sashay. She asks questions about my outfits, my relationships, my jewelry. I usually put one of the pieces on her to wear, moving the rings past her knobby knuckles. She looks at it and smiles, pretending to pose. She is also eager to share the stories about her life with a fresh set of ears. I imagine that her family members have heard these stories dozens of times and might be tired of them. I pull up a seat on her left side away from the cream-colored curtain, slightly dirtied by the hands that pull it repeatedly during the day to restore a semblance of privacy to the residents.

During our visits, Ms. Bobbie entertains me while I lotion her thin hands, paint her nails plum, and tweeze her chin hairs that have grown wiry in neglect. The maroon velvet photo album on her nightstand holds a lifetime's worth of memories and smells faintly of Shalimar perfume. As a traveling nurse, she had been afforded rights to travel during the Jim Crow era even though she is Black. She brags about the places she'd seen that her friends had never heard of. Ms. Bobbie has been to China and wishes she could show me the pearls she'd bought as evidence. They'd been sold to pay for her stay in the eldercare home. She tells me of the husband she'd run off with a gun once she found out he'd cheated on her. She shared her other divorces—four in total, with many lovers in between. While I brush her hair, Ms. Bobbie insists she was one of the first Black women to wear her hair in a French roll in the US, because she'd seen it in Paris. She's lived in twenty-six homes in Los Angeles and holds pride in integrating a couple of neighborhoods. "You shoulda seen their white faces when I walked out in my robe and curlers on Sunday mornings to fetch the paper." When asked about how many great-grandchildren she'd had, with a snort Ms. Bobbie replies, "Baby, I lost count."

While she is nearing the end of her life, she is also still full of it. Even though she often repeats stories, Ms. Bobbie's memory for detail remains sharp. Over the course of a year, I watch her health slowly decline. Her stories get shorter and she's lost interest in eating except for the oatmeal cream pies you find at the gas station that I sneak in to her. They are soft enough for her to chew without her teeth. Her interest in having her hair brushed and nails painted also wanes.

In what turns out to be our third-to-last visit, I roll her out to the small courtyard in a wheelchair to look at the orchids she loves. They are finally in bloom and Ms. Bobbie is in awe of their color—magenta in the middle, crowned in white. I ask her if her ninety-four years—almost ninety-five, she interjects to remind me—make some kind of sense to her. She's had such a complex life. Women of her age typically got married, stayed that way, didn't work, and had children. But Ms. Bobbie carved her own path. I hope for a magic quote to ease a deep-seated fear that I am still doing life wrong. Maybe I should have stayed at Legal Aid. Maybe I should have stayed married to Kip. Maybe I should have had some kids.

In her casual way, Ms. Bobbie says, "Baby, I ain't figured shit out. My life was so messy. And I wouldn't change a goddamned thing." She pauses, purses her lips, and moves her jaw back and forth, mashing up the oatmeal cream pie in her gums. "Boy, it's been one hell of a ride."

Three weeks later, I get a phone call from one of her daughters to tell me that Ms. Bobbie has had a cardiac event. I offer comfort to her daughter and tell her that I am available for updates if and when she'd like to give them. Privately, I dismiss it as a minor occurrence since Ms. Bobbie has navigated much more in her life and comes through with stories to tell about it. A few minutes later, reality sets in. Ms. Bobbie's wild ride will soon be ending. She dies a few days before her ninety-fifth birthday, an occasion for which she'd planned to wear a red sequined dress with her hair done up in a French roll.

I am honored to be invited as a guest to Ms. Bobbie's funeral. It is not unusual, as I grow close to my clients and their families during the dying process, but this one is different. I've never met any of Ms. Bobbie's family members—our service agreement was made over the phone, documents were signed electronically, and my visits with Ms. Bobbie were one-on-one. Just me and Ms. Bobbie. I know names and stories, but the only faces are old yellowed photographs of moments captured forty or fifty years ago. Being at her funeral, I can feel Ms. Bobbie there. Most of the people look similar, as many of them are related to her and each other. Her eulogy, delivered by her oldest grandson, is intimate and shares stories more absurd than the ones I've heard. It adds layers to the woman who fought to live on her own terms at a time when life was supposed to be a cookie cutter version of one. This is her legacy, and it is stunning. I weep silently in the last pew in gratitude for her example.

There is a societal myth of "having it all." It's the one that says we're supposed to have great jobs, which are also our life purpose and passion, visible abs, successful children, clean houses, doting spouses, and perfect eyebrows. But eyebrows get overplucked in the early 2000s and never quite grow back. Human beings can never be perfect. At some point, every last one of us will weaken, come apart, and die.

Many of us reach the end of life still ruminating on the things we believe we were "supposed" to do. But there is no guidebook to life. We just come in a sack of matter waiting for life to do what it will. Making peace with the phantom-life guidebook is a work many only do on the deathbed, when it's too late to correct course. While living, we can make a life that we can feel comfortable dying from.

I've spent so much of my life trying to untangle myself from the thicket of the expectations of others and unlearn the rules that society gave me about what life should be. Living my life in "supposed to" has brought me more pain than purpose and certainly more sadness than satisfaction. The question I ask myself second most often is still, "Am I doing this right?" (The first question is "Am I hungry or bored?")

The answer is always YES. I am hungry. And yes, I am doing it right. No matter what anyone else might be thinking. It is my life and I am the only one who will have to reckon with the choices I made on my deathbed.

We only know what kind of story it is once we know the ending, and we want a Hollywood ending. We want to wrap it all up with a shiny bow where there might be a steaming pile of shit. Life doesn't work that way. Death doesn't either. It can be tangled, torturous, fraught with surprises and hard left turns. That pretty bow to sit on top of a life might not come. It could be the wreath that sits atop a coffin.

All we know is that everything ends. Our collective death denial inspires us to behave like we can live forever. But we don't have forever to create the life we want.

For life's sake, don't die with a freezer full of bananas. Make the banana bread. Scream into the pillow. Take a nap. Eat the cake. Forgive yourself. Buy the shoes. Apologize to the people you've hurt. Watch the birds make a nest. Tell your truth. Tell the ones you love that you love them. Fuck. A lot. And make love. Quit the job. Or *take* the job. Whatever it is that *you* know you must do to reconcile your life with your death. Do it. Do it today. And don't stop until you get enough.

Glitter Wave

I think about my death almost every day. Sometimes it's because I am doing something kind of ridiculous like roller skating in the kitchen. I almost slip, and I imagine knocking myself out on the counter. Sometimes I think about my death because I've just stood at the gateway between this world and whatever comes next, witnessing the death of another. I still wonder how a human can have a spark of life in them, which then evaporates like a puff of smoke. And sometimes I think about my death because my entire life is leading up to that mystifying moment.

None of us knows what happens when life is over. Many of us understandably choose to fill that space of not knowing with dread, out of the fear of leaving the only place we have experienced. Yet, in our everyday lives, when we think about taking a trip someplace we've never been, we can anticipate it joyfully. We can do the same with our deaths, if we choose to, adding sensory detail so lush we can feel it in our bones.

Here is what *I* choose:

In the moments before my death, I am lying in my own bed, which is on a deck outside. My senses are fully engaged, to the extent my dying body can handle, since this is the last time they get to take in the sights, sounds, smells, and touch that I've come to treasure.

Allowing my eyes to feast on their last sunset, I want to see water-color oranges, luscious pinks, and vibrant purples as the day dies into night over the treetops. I want to hear the wind fluttering through the leaves while the trees sway in their decades-long synchronized dance. I only hear the quiet chatter of my loved ones and the sound of softly running water, from a creek just below.

Orange and yellow sunflowers surround me on the deck, along with some peonies, which I can still smell from my deathbed. Nag champa amber incense floats gently into my nostrils. I can also smell the trees and the dank, musty earth. My last meal hopefully included a fried ripe plantain, though my declining body likely hasn't wanted food for weeks.

My friends and family do not hover, but they keep an eye on me in case I say something memorable. With my luck and sailor's mouth, my last words will be "Holy fucking shit!"

A soft fleece blanket covers me, and I've got on cozy socks. I hate cold feet and shudder at the thought of that being one of my last earthly sensations. My lips are moisturized, as is my skin, because I've got caregivers who know that I don't go anywhere ashy, especially not into my death. Gotta keep my body looking as chocolatey as it can. And I better not be wearing a bra.

My affairs are wrapped up and my loved ones know what to do with my possessions and my remains: I want a green burial. Place my body directly into the earth, covered only by a hot-pink and orange raw silk burial shroud, no more than three and a half feet underground so the bugs can devour my cellulite and dispose of my body naturally. They also have instructions for my funeral. It must be outside with my jewelry decorating low-hanging tree branches. I want those in attendance to grab a piece and wear it home.

Brightly colored Gerbera daisies are on the tables, and photographs I've taken from my travels are all around.

I want my mourners to wear an outfit they feel like their most fabulous selves in, and to drink a whole lot of tequila, to dance, to cry, to sing, to laugh, and to comfort each other.

I've left my beloveds with one most important directive: to tell the truth about who I am. Honor the richness of my lived experience for what it is—a blink of time in a pinprick of a body on a speck of a planet in a vast, vast universe. I want them to acknowledge the hugeness and the tininess of this.

I hope my loved ones say that I lived in love and that I did my work. I want them to say that I encouraged them to stretch themselves into the edges of their lives and that I was not stingy. They better not make me a saint. I am just as equally a sinner. I want them to feel proud that they gave me the grace to be human, and I want them to acknowledge when I was not the best version of myself. I reserve the right to change my mind, to acknowledge my mistakes, to shift my beliefs, and to grow until my death. I can be generous, loving, intuitive, purposeful, bold, and goofy. But I can also be righteous, petty, greedy, stubborn, judgmental, and impulsive. I'm a whole person.

I want to die safe: safe in body but also safe in my being, free to express discomfort and fear when it arises; safe in the knowledge that my loved ones will hold me there. They feel safe too. They speak freely with me about their grief over my impending death and allow me to feel my own grief about leaving. My tears fall without a need to wipe them away. And if I haven't learned it before, at my deathbed, I will feel no shame about the depths of my emotions.

I might be scared to leave behind everything I have ever known and loved, but I'm also ready. At my death, I am devoid of every last ounce of skill and talent I have cultivated. I am, finally, used up.

I want to die in gratitude. I've moved fast my entire life, yet I want to saunter into my death like a tipsy woman might walk to a lover across a dark room. I go in surrender.

All of my questions about my life are over. No more concerns about whether I was good enough to be loved as I am. I know that I was.

No more worry about what others think about the choices I made. Any doubts I had about how I used my time are vanquished.

My ongoing struggles with depression, doubt, and impulses toward mayhem have finally ended. I can no longer run away from the burdens I've created. It is done.

My body, in its perfect size and ability, carried me through this life and I'm now at the moment of its death. It knows how to die.

My breathing has slowed down significantly, and my heart, weakened, is doing its best to pump blood to failing organs. My central nervous system has also slowed, yet the system of nerves, veins, and arteries that map my body start to tingle, as all of the dopamine, serotonin, DMT, and other feel-good chemicals course through me. I'd always wondered if dying feels bad, but in fact this feels good.

My sensory experience is growing thin, but inside my body, all of the sensations and emotions I experienced while living are starting to gather up. Slowly crescendo-ing, I begin to feel every joy, sorrow, excitement, grief, embarrassment, orgasm, shame, freedom, guilt, and glee that I have ever felt. I also feel the little things, like the squish of a frog I stepped on in Nairobi under my bare feet, the rising heat in a car after the windows have been closed on a summer day, and the opening notes to Stevie Wonder's "As." Most prominently, I feel love in its aching beauty. Love for myself, for my imperfect life, and for the humans, animals, plants, and insects that journeyed alongside me. This is it.

I've lost connection to the outside world, as my consciousness starts to swirl inside my body and move toward my heart center. My loved ones who have gathered to hold vigil hang on to my every breath. They do not have to wait long, as I release one final, soft exhale. My lungs rest and my body reverts to matter.

Following my instructions, my beloveds clap, in celebration of the life I loved and the grace with which I let it go. But I can only hear them very faintly. My senses have dulled.

My consciousness expands outward, past the edges of my body, which can no longer contain the depth and breadth of my human experience. It is no longer responding to external stimuli or perceiving myself as separate from others. As the cells inside my body die, my consciousness expands bigger and bigger like a helium balloon. I am beginning to experience the freedom of death. The freedom in not knowing and enjoying the ride anyway. Just when I've felt every single sensation my human body has ever felt and cannot take another instant, the "I," as I know myself, bursts into a firework of brightly colored, glittery confetti. It fills the atmosphere with flecks of every conceivable color.

When the confetti reaches its apex, having been hurled into the atmosphere with the impact of my life force, it scatters slowly, like soft snow. These pieces of confetti represent who I was as a human, as I am an amalgamation of everyone I have ever met and every experience I've ever had. The pieces of confetti land in greater concentration on the people who loved me, and in lesser concentration on the people whose lives I touched. It will cling to them just like glitter does, getting stuck in every crevice of their being. This is how our dead stay with us.

In these flecks of glitter falling from the ether, I can see my dad eating the cardboard veggie burger and my mom hot-glueing stars onto my Burning Man boots. Those are gold pieces of glitter.

I see six-year-old Bozoma hiding under the table while the "Thriller" video plays, and Ahoba cute and pregnant with my nephew Jahcir. I also see his feet, which grew before my eyes from pudgy, dimply stumps to a size 13. They are bronze, red, and navy.

Aba's thoughtful and caring nature twinkles through, in rose-colored bits of confetti.

I see Kip's big ole smile in blue glitter flakes.

In yellow, I see my friends and former partners—the laughs we shared, the mirrors we held up, and the pain we carried for each other.

Looking up and around, I see Ms. Bobbie eating her oatmeal cream pies, Ken's gold skirt, Tash's teeny-weeny gap in her teeth, Nancy's hair barrettes. I see Jack's love for his sons, Justina's Pomeranians, Dora's work plaques, James's baby mamas, Summer's baptism, Akua's dancing arms, and Leslie's decorative spoons—all represented in sparkles of colorful confetti. And many, many others.

All around, I see Peter. Everywhere. I see his love of the Ghanaian condiment shito that he puts on everything, as well as his cool leather jackets. I see him throwing Lael into the air and see her delight in orange confetti. I see his inability to turn down any challenge I suggest and his love of Boston sports teams. Those flecks are turquoise. But in deep magenta, I see the pain his death caused and the hole I carried throughout my life in his absence.

All of the little pieces of me that didn't stick with anyone, like my secrets and old hair bonnets, drift down and gently crash into each other in a massive wave of glitter. Big swells of the brightest and most vibrant colors undulate across eternity as far as I can sense, moving to a rhythm as familiar as my walking gait.

Slowly, the pieces of glitter confetti that once made up the magically mundane earthly experiences of Alua Adwoba Arthur are seamlessly enveloped back into the wave. Even the littlest pieces get swallowed and gobbled up, becoming part of that grand cosmic expanse once again. And "I" am no more.

I have returned to all that ever was and all that ever will be. It is complete. And I am safe.

There is joy.

There is peace.

There is rapture.

There is pure, abiding love.

There was my individual life, now extinguished, and indistinguishable from the billions who have come before and will die after.

This is my hope for when I die.

I hope death feels like riding a bright glitter wave, but I don't know. And since I don't know if I'll have it in my death, I will make it with my life. I look for the glitter in everything.

We can spend our lives fretting about our deaths, or we can use our brief time to sink deeper into the experience of being human, for all it entails. The good, the tricky, the impermanent. We can acknowledge that our death will one day come and use that knowledge to create a life so whole, so honest, so juicy, that it is worth leaving. I have seen over and over human beings' personal reckonings in the final moments of life. It begs the question: What must I do to be at peace with myself so that I may live presently and die gracefully?

Without our deaths, none of it would matter. There would be no context for what we do. When we live in relationship to our mortality, it adds direction to our actions, truth to our words, rapture to our experience, authenticity to our being, and maybe pounds to our hips. We can make choices that resonate with the core of our being, free from societal expectations and the judgments of others.

While our lives and choices may seem insignificant in the grand scheme of things, they are not. With the dizzying serendipity that must occur for us to be born, the fact that we live is a miracle. If the best that we do on any given day is roll over in bed—so long as we make peace with our choices from the perspective of our deaths—there is cause to celebrate. A daily practice of being with mortality gives us the glorious opportunity to refine our priorities, redefine our values, and bring wonder and mystery to this wild ride of our unique lives. This allows us to reach the end downright raggedy, satiated, and drunk on life—but ready to go home 'cause the party is over and our feet hurt.

This is what I wish for all of us: a life that feels like the miracle it is and a death that serves as a period on a satisfying sentence. *Because we live, we get to die.* That is a gift.

Acknowledgments

Writing a book is both a death and a birth. The book itself labored to be born and parts of me, the writer, had to die for it to do so. I got vulnerable and intimate with my life and just as with many deaths, I resisted, got angry, tried everything but accepting the reality, then eventually surrendered—like we all must do. Here are the people who saw me, sat vigil, and told me I was doing it right. They doula'd me and the book. Please forgive me if I haven't named you. Your love was still felt.

First and foremost, thank you to my family: Dr. Appianda Arthur, Aba Enim, Bozoma Saint John, Dr. Ahoba Arthur, Aba Arthur, Peter Saint John, Lael Saint John, and Jahcir Murphy. You are a source of constant inspiration, laughter, and a reminder about what I'm made of when I forget. I'm sorry for wishing you were a boy, Aba. I am so grateful you are exactly who you became.

To thirteen-year-old Alua, wearing braids while riding her Marvin the Martian skateboard through the white neighborhood to start a recycling program, and who kept going door to door, when many opened and then were shut, without getting a single can: thank you for continuing to ride. Thank you for staying true to yourself the very best that you could. It's still a little bumpy, but we're doing alright, even if we're no longer riding a skateboard 'cause I want to preserve our kneecaps.

Thank you to my editor, Rakia Clark, for championing my vision, working tirelessly to make it see the light, for your T-shirt with my face on it, for holding space for my messiness, for despising split infinitives. To Lindsey Kennedy and Tavia Kowalchuk, who, with Rakia, fiercely carried this book in their hearts and into rooms where it needed to be seen. To Mark Robinson, for this bomb-ass cover. To the entire team at Mariner Books, for believing that this first-time writer could pull it off. To my agent, Anna Sproul-Latimer, who held my hand, listened to me vent, answered all of my real questions and sent me right back to myself for the answers only I held. To Jayson Greene, who got in the trench with me to complete this book and made me a better writer and a more compassionate human. To Kim Green, who coached and coaxed out the very first iteration of this book. Kim is the first person who said, "I think you got something here!"

To the core team at Going with Grace, who kept the business thriving while I stepped away and into myself to complete this book: Aba (again), Alica Forneret, Sara Westfall, Tracey Walker, Corie McMillan, Nicole Briggs-Gary, Valenca Valenzuela, and Shannon Kranzler. Your dedication, passion, attention to excellence, and the reminder about "why" buoyed me. Baxley Andresen: you get infinite purple hearts. To Corinne Bowen and Corinne Consulting, thank you for the space to play with my ideas to see which we could make a reality. To Emily Marquez—aka Emerald Fields Forever—I would have been lost without you. Thank you for making space for the business to become what it is.

To the students of the Going with Grace End of Life Training course and the past student guides: Wow. You are the realest—the most provocative, thoughtful, hilarious, and creative folks I know. You call me up into more precise iterations of the work.

To Annie Georgia Greenberg: When I struggled with sharing myself widely for Refinery29, you reminded me that people hear the message because of the messenger's story. If not for that strong nudge, I never would have done this.

To the death and dying community: We are all the messengers. I am honored to be in your ranks. In particular, thank you to Dr. B. J. Miller, Caitlin Doughty, Claire Bidwell Smith, Lashanna Williams, Michelle Acciavatti, E. E. Miller, Katrina Spade, Elizabeth Erbrecht, Narinder Bazen, Dr. Shoshana Ungerleider, and Tembi Locke for not taking any of this too seriously and for holding life lightly. Olivia Bareham: you are a trailblazer and my forever teacher.

To all of the folks who paved the way by talking and writing about how we die long before it was cool, I am filled with gratitude.

To LP123: You are shining examples of leadership and no quit. Thank you for holding me. Jessica Blue: your humor, authenticity, and faith in me over the years have been invaluable. Margo Majdi: You told me to write a book five years before I conceived of it and expanded what I now know I am capable of. I am eternally grateful for your coaching even in your final act. Rest in love.

To my Legal Aid friends who offered a haven when all felt like it was going to shit: Ji-lan Zang, Carolina Sheinfeld, Vanessa Lee—you kept me alive with pastries and laughter. Malcolm Carson, Karla Barrow, Debra Sudo-Marr, Joe Kotzin, and all the Legal Aiders who made the unbearable bearable. Silvia Argueta, you were right. Going to Inglewood Self-Help, aka The Dungeon, was the very best thing that happened to me.

To my many friends who listened to me talk incessantly about the struggles to navigate this process: we did it!! A special thank you to my lifers: Magda Labonté-Blaise, Kim Velez, Richard Frank, Aurora Colindres, Anastasia Baranova, Jessica Amisial, Dr. Kwame Ohemeng, Patima Komolamit, my sister-cousins Joanne Sogbaka and Dorien Agyapon, Breeda Desmond, Folake Ologunja, Brookelin Barnhill, Ariane Aumont, Allison Kunath, Jacqui Ruiz, and my law school and forever buddies Kristin Bowers Tompkins, Rachel MacGuire, Jess Curtis, Jenni Cohen. To my book writing crew: Carla Fernandez, Scott Shigeoka, Liz Tran, you are superstars.

To mah kumah toffee, my heart's candy, my safest space: Thank you will never be enough. You make me smile with all my teeth and pour love into even the parts of me that I do not want anyone to see and believe are difficult to love. You balance me, ground me, pull me back from doubt, and make my belly flip when you walk in the door or I smell your shirt. I hope you always know that I love you with every fiber of my being. Thank you for never getting tired of talking about death.

To every person who offered me a stage or a simple "your work matters," you keep me going. To the clients who shared their lives with me, you all doula'd me into new versions of myself and a greater acceptance of the glorious weirdness of life and the power of a single human story.

I also just gotta thank this book. To *Briefly Perfectly Human*: Thank you for laboring to be born, for forcing my hand at surrender, for teaching me about dying. You kicked my ass. Thank you for pushing me through fear and for showing me the way. I am grateful that you allowed me to be your steward.

To the reader: Thank you for allowing me to share my life and my deaths with you. Thank you for allowing me to be human.

ABOUT
MARINER BOOKS

Mariner Books traces its beginnings to 1832 when William Ticknor cofounded the Old Corner Bookstore in Boston, from which he would run the legendary firm Ticknor and Fields, publisher of Ralph Waldo Emerson, Harriet Beecher Stowe, Nathaniel Hawthorne, and Henry David Thoreau. Following Ticknor's death, Henry Oscar Houghton acquired Ticknor and Fields and, in 1880, formed Houghton Mifflin, which later merged with venerable Harcourt Publishing to form Houghton Mifflin Harcourt. HarperCollins purchased HMH's trade publishing business in 2021 and reestablished their storied lists and editorial team under the name Mariner Books.

Uniting the legacies of Houghton Mifflin, Harcourt Brace, and Ticknor and Fields, Mariner Books continues one of the great traditions in American bookselling. Our imprints have introduced an incomparable roster of enduring classics, including Hawthorne's *The Scarlet Letter*, Thoreau's *Walden*, Willa Cather's *O Pioneers!*, Virginia Woolf's *To the Lighthouse*, W.E.B. Du Bois's *Black Reconstruction*, J.R.R. Tolkien's *The Lord of the Rings*, Carson McCullers's *The Heart Is a Lonely Hunter*, Ann Petry's *The Narrows*, George Orwell's *Animal Farm* and *Nineteen Eighty-Four*, Rachel Carson's *Silent Spring*, Margaret Walker's *Jubilee*, Italo Calvino's *Invisible Cities*, Alice Walker's *The Color Purple*, Margaret Atwood's *The Handmaid's Tale*, Tim O'Brien's *The Things They Carried*, Philip Roth's *The Plot Against America*, Jhumpa Lahiri's *Interpreter of Maladies*, and many others. Today Mariner Books remains proudly committed to the craft of fine publishing established nearly two centuries ago at the Old Corner Bookstore.